Tactical Development for Beginners

A Guide to Becoming Dangerous

Jonathan Von Moltke

Copyright © 2024

All Rights Reserved

No part of this book may be reproduced or transmitted in any form or by any means, electronic or mechanical, including photocopying, recording, or by any information storage and retrieval system without the written permission of the author, except where permitted by law.

ISBN: 978-1-917096-40-9

Table of Contents

What Does Being Dangerous Mean?... 1

Are You Easy to Kill? 4

Physical Readiness 8

Mental Toughness... 12

Skills vs. Tactics.. 17

Everyday Carry (EDC) Essentials 19

Danger/ Target Zones to Avoid 28

Proper Training 32

"Fire Drills" 36

Ethics vs. Morals... 39

Is The Juice Worth the Squeeze?.. 41

Observe, Orient, Decide, Act 44

Risk Mitigation 48

Reticular Activating System (RAS)... 57

The Fundamentals of Marksmanship 61

Quick and Easy Skills and Tactics.. 67

Basic CQB Principles and Tactics.. 76

Recommended Combat Drills 85

Basic Spontaneous Knife Defense 88

Reacting to an Active Shooter 92

Basic Self-Defense Tactics 99

The Zombie Apocalypse – The Final Test 109

Conclusion 114

About the Author 115

What Does Being Dangerous Mean?

Being dangerous is a concept that essentially means that you have a strong desire to live. In today's world, statistics show that the average American is likely to be the victim of a violent crime at some point in their life. As someone with a strong desire to live, the need to be proactive in your defense capabilities grows as the world becomes a riskier place to live in. Many places are more dangerous to live in than the United States; however, many people from other countries do not appear "dangerous" Consider this: If a person was raised in a third-world country having to fend for themselves, protect their family from rampant gangs and cartels, survive daily violence, and endure government overreach, would that person appear to be dangerous in a first-world country simply due to their culture and experiences?

Much of what we consider to be cultural differences are humans' adaptation to their environment, becoming situationally dangerous. For example, many hobbyists in the United States like to practice survival skills by going camping with limited resources, foraging for food, hunting, building fires, and facing the elements. To a person who lives in the Amazon, this is every day. To them, they don't consider themselves to be expert survivalists but instead, normal people who live like everyone else.

To be dangerous is to break out of the normal for what surrounds you and become comfortable with discomfort. It's physical readiness, technological proficiency, mental toughness, and the ability to analyze risk and adapt accordingly, using discipline and speed. In a crowded room, the most dangerous person is the one who is most knowledgeable and comfortable with violence and the most capable of violent actions. They're the person who can identify the largest risk and quickly strategize how to address that risk should the need arise.

Proactivity in response to risk doesn't have to exist to be dangerous. Many apex predators are ambush animals, waiting for the right time to strike. In fact, most venomous animals will not proactively pursue prey. However, they are considered some of the most dangerous. Many people would prefer to deal with an angry dog than a rattlesnake, even though the dog can do more immediate physical damage, potentially chase you, and has a higher level of intelligence. It's because, in the back of your mind, you know that a bite from a dog is less likely to kill you than one from a rattlesnake. Being dangerous is about playing to your strengths. It's about maximizing your capabilities without spending time and effort in areas that will not help you in a violent situation.

This book is for those with no tactical experience who want to be better. This book is here to teach you what it really takes to be optimized in the face of danger. There are thousands of different ways to accomplish this elusive task, and this book describes my opinions based on my knowledge and experiences. If you don't agree with what is written here, that is your choice. However, I offer you a perspective that will probably be different from every other tactic-cool operator you have watched on YouTube with information that has been physically demonstrated in real life.

Are You Easy to Kill?

Yes. Unfortunately, humans are easy to kill, and this statement is supported by science. Having lived in a civilized society for generations, humans have evolved to no longer need protection from elements, starvation, predators, and violence from other beings. While all these situations still cause death to humans, it is not a common occurrence to most people due to the society we have built and currently live in daily.

If we look at nature as a spectrum, we can see perfect examples that support these statements. Alligators have armor-like scales protecting them from attacks from other predators while also allowing them to be agile in water and mud, where they thrive the most. Bears have thick fur to keep them warm and large claws to climb trees, scoop fish from water, and protect them from danger. Sharks have white bellies to camouflage them while they circle prey from above, while dart frogs have bright coloration to warn potential predators of their toxicity. Snakes with the most potent venom typically use the smallest amounts of venom per bite because they have evolved to be more efficient. When we look at evidence of cavemen and their physical features, we will discover they were very hairy people. Much like fur, this kept them warm and protected them from harsh winds, disease-carrying insects, and even minor cuts and scrapes that could not be treated for infections.

Currently, humans are much different than the cavemen era. We have little hair on our bodies, we are generally weaker, and mentally unprepared for potential dangers in nature. We do not have the biological need to camouflage ourselves due to a lack of any natural predators.

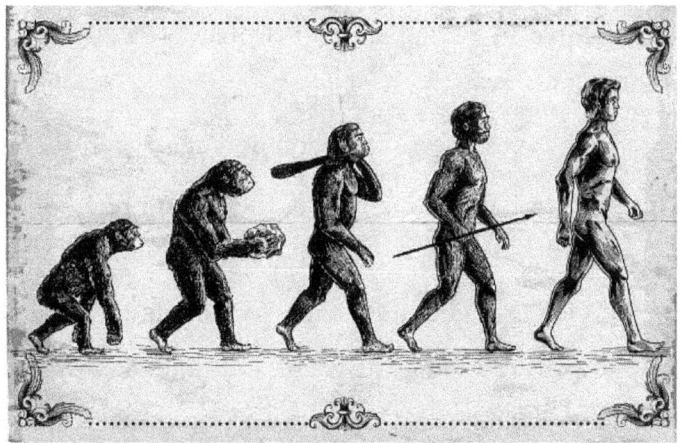

Humans are the most intelligent species on earth, growing more intelligent with every generation. This trend causes us to continue finding solutions to problems and eliminating the need for primitive skills. Even within our lifetime, we have found solutions that we did not think would be possible a mere 20 years ago. I recall in school that my teacher assigned us math equations, and enjoyed reminding us that we would not always have a calculator in our pocket to solve it for us. Enter 2023, where it isn't unusual for a first-grade child to own and carry a smartphone.

We are easy to kill because we have created generational vulnerabilities due to evolution, innovative technology, societal norms, and cultural support. Our vital organs are unprotected, and clothing does little to shield us from injury. Our schools teach academia and not survival. Less than 10% of our nation has participated in a combat sport or martial art. That leaves over 200 million Americans clueless of violence, survival, and danger. That leaves over 200 million potential victims.

Consider that in the real world, there is no referee. There are no rules, and there is no such thing as fighting dirty. Many victims of violent crimes are unable to identify their attackers because they were caught off guard and they didn't see what their assailant looked like. Criminals are opportunists and have constantly demonstrated that they will take any advantage they can in violent confrontations. They have attacked the weak, robbed the elderly, and used firearms, bombs, vehicles and other weapons of opportunity against large crowds in a defenseless populous. There is no honor in real-world violence, and unfair practices are not recognized. People are easy to kill because they choose to ignore these criminals. They purposefully remain ignorant to the violence that may be happening right under their noses. They avoid confrontation in all forms, including political, physical, and mental. This causes us to not only become complacent but unprepared for the likelihood that we will one day be victimized. If you choose to dismiss the fact that car accidents happen every single day, you will be less inclined to wear a seatbelt.

Physical Readiness

Pop culture forces us to believe that a dangerous person must have washboard abs, chiseled pectoral muscles, and budging vascular biceps. I mean, how could you possibly defend yourself without traps that touch your ears or a back that resembles a cloud, right? Honestly, having muscles has nothing to do with being physically prepared for danger. Being in good shape is always beneficial to overall wellness and reacting to violence, but is by no means a requirement. Many people are unable to exercise due to medical restraints, financial situations, or mental barriers. These same individuals have the capacity to be dangerous. Understanding the difference between strength and aesthetics is important, just as understanding that owning a gun and being able to operate one proficiently are two different things.

Being physically ready requires you to assess your situation and customize your readiness based on the elements that you determine would likely be a factor in a dangerous scenario. For example, if you live on the 17th floor of an apartment building and following the philosophy that we will always choose to avoid confrontation first, you may have to use a fire escape to leave. This means that physically, you should be able to quickly navigate 17 flights of stairs, based on the needs of your situation. If I live in a single-story rancher, I will more than likely not have to be able to navigate 17 flights of stairs, but maybe I'll have to be able to push open heavy cellar doors to leave the house. If I have spent time becoming proficient in a martial art, such as judo, BJJ, or karate, and I plan on making that an element of my response, I need to ensure that I am physically able to use it as the years progress. You can't depend on a fire extinguisher that hasn't been certified for 15 years. If you were a black belt in karate in your junior year of high school but haven't used it in 15 years, it probably isn't a realistic tool for you to depend on to secure your survival.

Tailoring your physical readiness doesn't have to be black and white and doesn't have to be a chore. A good practice is to mix up your training to include fun experiences that also promote physical development. If my exit strategy calls for me to be able to navigate 17 flights of stairs, maybe I can start hiking, or travel around to national monuments while only using stairs. This way, you're getting experiences that will make the "work" worth it in real time. Be creative in your approach to readiness, and you may find that it comes easier than you thought it would. When most people think of fitness, they imagine themselves in a hot gym, sweating and listening to loud music while going to battle with themselves mentally. They think of gritting their teeth and pushing for one more rep until exhaustion finally wins, and they can go home feeling accomplished while simultaneously dreading doing the same thing tomorrow. Fitness doesn't have to be a battle. Having an active lifestyle can be enjoyable and give you all the exercise you need to accomplish the required goals in your situation. Don't be discouraged if you're not a triathlete; being dangerous is about much more than just fitness.

Another consideration in your physical fitness is your diet. Much like exercise (and against increasingly popular opinion), you don't have to always eat "clean" to be adequately fit. A diet doesn't have to be a life-changing experience that lasts forever and eliminates your favorite foods. Again, consider your personal requirements and tailor them accordingly. If you love pizza, consider eating two slices instead of your normal four. Maybe switch to diet soda instead of drinking the full unleaded version. It'll taste odd at first, but in two days, it'll be normal, and you will be fine with it.

Moderation is all you need to take the first step in physical readiness. Don't get caught up in the noise of modern fitness influencers telling you that you must be a caffeine-addicted gym rat to be healthy. You do not have to weigh your food for every meal, you don't have to go vegan, you don't have to eat 250 grams of protein a day, and you don't have to trash your social life. Drink water, eat three appropriately sized meals a day, and be active throughout the day as much as you can. That's the answer to the equation. You may even find that the relaxation of your obnoxious diet (which has failed 313 times in the last two years) lowers your stress level and causes you to trim a few pounds. Ironic, right?

Mental Toughness

One of the most powerful tools in your arsenal is mental strength. In Basic Training for the U.S. Army, the mental factor was more difficult to overcome than anything else. Sure, the physical requirements were rigorous, the sleep deprivation was hard, and I truly loathed working 6 days a week, but the mental stress was the biggest thorn in my side. They dress all of you alike and shave your hair off, taking away your individualism and molding you into a copy of everyone around you. You get disciplined for everyone else's mistakes, and there is no grievance process to fall back on should you not like a decision. You have no contact with your loved ones for months. No social media, no phone, no sugar in your diet, and insufficient food to counter all the exercises you had to do as a discipline. You weren't given the option of a rebuttal. If a drill sergeant said something, that word was law, regardless of whether it was fair. Mentally, you were broken down to the lowest place you could go.

At a certain point in my training, things started to shift. The drill sergeants would surprise you with an extra 5 minutes of sleep or give everyone a two-minute phone call home. While this doesn't sound much, it was more valuable than gold. We would be informed that these actions were rewards for doing well, and it made us want to be better and push ourselves harder to earn the rewards on the other end of the equation. They broke us down to nothing and built us into motivation machines. We enjoyed being forced to exercise because we knew it would strengthen us. We enjoyed eating no sugar and little food because it would allow us to lose weight and run longer. We appreciated not getting to talk to our friends and family because we knew that we would not be here forever and wanted to take advantage of this training opportunity.

Our mindset was armored, and our wills were strengthened. Our "Soldiers Creed" offers the words "I will never quit." This was our bread and butter. Against all odds, even when you know for a fact you will lose, you continue to drive on and adapt to the situation. If I die, they are going to feel me in their bones tomorrow. I will not stop running until I finish or pass out. I will figure out this problem even if I must stay here all night. Some call it stubbornness, we call it mental fortitude.

Applying this concept to the civilian world was not as easy as I thought. Working in law enforcement meant I was tasked with dealing with the public. Often, the public was weak minded and did not share the same standards that I did. It's a hard pill to swallow when you have been broken down and reborn as a problem solver, just to be told that some problem can't be fixed. I found myself at social outings with friends or visiting with my family, and remembering their conversations about problems they were dealing with annoyed me. If you're unemployed, go get a job instead of sitting here crying about it. If your partner left you, date someone else; you're probably better off now. I didn't understand how to transition from such a strict and structured mindset into a flexible one with contingencies. Ironically, I had trouble fixing my problem. Even though I was mentally tougher than I had ever been, I couldn't tailor my mind to the situations I hadn't prepared for. Your goal is to find a happy medium. Learn to apply that desire to win and will to live in dynamic situations while maintaining flexibility in your personal life. Some exercises can help you in this learning experience. Try sticking to a goal for a certain period and prioritize it above everything else. Start small and make the goal reasonable and realistic based on your schedule, finances, and capability. For example, you may try setting a goal of making your bed every day for a whole month. It sounds simple enough, but you will realize it can be a burden. You'll inevitably wake up one of those days and realize you're running late. Pause and stick to your goal. If you are 10 minutes late, is being 15 minutes late that much worse? Make your bed, then go. Maybe set a goal of doing 100 pushups every night for 30 days. It doesn't matter how long it takes you to do it, but make sure it's done every night. Stick to it and see how accomplished you feel after completing the goal. Use that motivation for your next goal.

Through this process, you will discipline your mind to stick to your goals and finish what you started. This also plays a part in staying alive. The desire to live has kept people alive in some of the worst situations imaginable. From patients being shot in the chest and surviving after being clinically dead, to a mother lifting a car off her baby who was run over, to people waking from a years-long coma. Unexplainable medically, but later interviews with these people revealed their will to live. They'll often say things like, "I couldn't leave my family behind yet," or "I still have much to offer this world."

Having that goal in mind and the discipline and desire to achieve it kept them alive. Picture the will to live as a big red button in a glass box that lives in the core of your brain. Once that button is pushed, you enter survival mode and take any steps necessary to continue living. This button doesn't get pushed often but is there when you need it. Typically, you can solve problems, even emergent ones, without pushing the button. However, when the shit hits the fan, that button is your hail-Mary. Tailoring your mind armor around the idea that you have a hidden contingency could prove to be a vital role in your life-saving efforts. There is always something else; you can't give up now.

Skills vs. Tactics

While this topic may sound confusing, it's important to understand the difference between skills and tactics, and how to train for them appropriately. A skill is something that takes time and effort to perfect. Hundreds of repetitions, muscle memory, and a singular focus to obtain a small progression of a particular skill. A tactic is a general process. Tactics are fluid and don't necessarily require a high skill level to use. For example, a skill would be going to the gun range and shooting the bullseye on a target with tight groups. Continuously shooting this way can make you very accurate and consistent and will certainly make you a better marksman (if your goal is marksmanship). Tactics, however, would be using a firearm to clear a building maintaining firearm fundamentals while safety navigating a structure. Clearing a building includes using angles and movement to remove a dwelling effectively from threats and danger. Every building is different and contains different furniture, layouts, and elements that require different tactics to clear.

I separate skills and tactics training into two groups: singular and value training. Singular training is a method used for a particular skill, focusing on a singular movement or action to achieve mastery. Value training is a method that is used to gain a fundamental understanding of a process and doesn't require mastery of a specific skill. Both methods are important for being dangerous, but they have different functions for which they are best used. Singular training can be shooting paper, reloading a firearm, sharpening a knife, or learning a specific martial art. Value training can be learning close-quarters battle (CQB) methods for tactical movement, shooting on the move, spontaneous knife defense, and learning a blend of multiple combat disciplines to understand the human body and how to manipulate it.

Applying the process to practice, you may decide that your efforts are best used to focus on a singular task. Maybe you work from home, live in a studio apartment, and have one firearm. In this situation, you are more inclined to experience a dangerous incident at home. Therefore, training to react to a threat at the entrance to your home may be the most important form of training you can do. On the other hand, if you work in a retail store in a large city, there are countless possibilities for encountering danger; therefore, value training in general threat reaction may be more suitable to your needs.

Everyday Carry (EDC) Essentials

Aligning with the other chapters in this book, the gear you choose to have at any given time should be tailored to your specific needs and situation. Everyone has different elements to their lives, and choosing gear is very similar to choosing other things such as clothing, vehicles, and home locations. What are your specific needs, and how does your everyday carry (EDC) gear need to support you? There are thousands and thousands of different "essential" gear options on the consumer market right now. Honestly, it's become a bit of a "Barbie-style" accessory market. Barbie has her friends, her car, her dream house, her Malibu estate, her specialized clothing, her career accessories, and an endless line of gear. Now put practice into play: a dangerous person has the training, firearms, clothing, vehicle accessories, bags, knives, survival gear, and the list goes on and on. The reality, however, will slap you in the face when you spend a year's salary on all the latest gear just to find that you can't carry it all, you don't use half of it, and there is already a newer, better product on the market.

You've undoubtedly heard it before: "Keep it simple, stupid" (KISS). This is a great philosophy (in moderation) regarding EDC. You're running to the grocery store to pick up some milk and bread; do you really need a foldable rifle, 6 full magazines, a complete medical kit, 3 knives, combat boots, 2 fire starters, and a satellite phone? Probably not. At the same time, it's easy to play 'what if', the unsullied truth is that you will more than likely never use the gear that you buy. Moderation can be your best friend. Instead of buying the $4,000 2011 pistol with the $800 RMR optic, the $200 competition grade IWB holster with the side car, and 4 extra $70 magazines, maybe consider buying a $500 Glock 19 with a decent $75 holster. Just because you want to wear a seatbelt doesn't mean it needs a red one found inside of a Ferrari (unless you're just into that sort of thing).

So, what do you need when it comes to EDC? I believe there are some core elements to EDC that I will always use as the foundation for my gear loadout.

1. A quality handgun with 1 extra magazine.
2. A quality knife
3. A flashlight.
4. A cell phone.
5. A tourniquet.

Let's get into it. A quality handgun means a gun that you will trust your life to. Remembering the KISS philosophy, we don't need an expensive gun for it to be good quality. Go to the gun range and try out a few options until you find one you are comfortable with. Watch unboxing and testing videos on YouTube and see what matches your specific needs. Finally, buy it and practice with it. I have multiple different options that I use for EDC, and I have thousands of rounds through each one of them. I want to know that my seatbelt will work properly during a collision, and I can confidently say that for all my EDC handguns.

A quality knife is important for multiple reasons. Quality means a good, durable steel that is corrosion resistant, can hold an edge, and doesn't cost a fortune. I prefer to use steel like 3V, S30V, M390, or even 5120 carbon steel from reputable companies. First, you never know when you're going to need to use a knife in self-defense. While it isn't pretty to imagine, you may find yourself in a close-quarters situation where a firearm isn't the best option. Having a good knife that you know how to use can save your life where a firearm would fail. Second, you may need a knife for a utility purpose, such as cutting a seatbelt to free you from a car, or to open emergency supplies in the heat of the moment. Hell, you may just need a knife to open your mail, but it's better to have it and not need it than to… well, you get the idea. A knife is one of the most essential pieces of gear you can have; however, if you plan to use it as a self-defense tool, you *must* train with it. Most defensive knives also have a similar training version available. I have recently purchased a Clinch Pick from Shivworks. When I made this purchase, I also purchased the training version with no edge. I have practiced carrying it, deploying it, and using it for months before adding it to my EDC options. It's important to understand that wearing unfamiliar gear is the equivalent of making a speech in public without preparing anything; you aren't certain how it will go, and it usually turns out sloppy. Regarding my life, I'd rather be certain, confident, and prepared.

A flashlight is an often-overlooked piece of equipment that you won't think about needing until you're inevitably in the dark at some point. While it may seem nifty to have an app on your smartphone that has a flashlight, the hard truth is that it is not powerful enough to do anything for you short of finding your wallet that fell between the seats in your car. A small flashlight with a high lumen count and a pocket clip can truly save you from a situation where you would otherwise be in the dark (pun intended). There are plenty of good options for quality flashlights on the market today. Streamlight, Surefire, Olight, and Stinger are good options to get you looking in the right direction. Make sure it is small enough to be carried comfortably in your pocket, has an LED light, and is durable.

Cell phones on an EDC list would cause people to scratch their heads, mainly because it's something that most people carry every day anyway. Considering how many people utilize technology, though, it may surprise you to know that many substitute their phones for things like a watch or an app on their laptop. Something to understand is that it's easier to call the police than it is to text 911. Though it's possible in many jurisdictions, it is commonly followed by a phone call anyway. Being able to use your phone to call in an emergency in a dynamic situation is critical and would be very difficult to accomplish on a watch or laptop.

Finally, a tourniquet (TQ) is something that I personally carry every day. You may find that it doesn't fit your daily loadout philosophy, and that's okay. I have trained with multiple different tourniquets, and I own several different holsters for my TQ that allow me to carry one without much hassle. In my opinion, carrying a TQ is a no-brainer. Specifically, I know that I may need to use a TQ on myself or my family in a defensive situation. I also know that controlling bleeding is statistically one of the best ways to increase the likelihood of survival after a dynamic incident. A few honorable mentions that seem to be a good idea in theory but did not make my fundamental list are:

1. Rifle
2. Go Bag/Get Home Bag
3. Food/Water Supply

Of course, I love the idea of having a rifle in a chaotic situation. A rifle is a true battle tool that may change the pace of a dynamic situation and potentially save a life. So why not add it to a fundamentals list? I did not add a rifle because I believe that EDC truly means every day. If I leave the house for any reason, I have my EDC loadout. This means if I go to a family barbeque if I go to the grocery store, if I go to a park with my family, I have this gear. It is unreasonable to honestly believe that I will bring a rifle with me to all these functions. Popping a pistol in a holster and a knife in my pocket is a quick function compared to stowing a full rifle setup in my vehicle in an inconspicuous manner. Instead, I fall back on my military and law enforcement training that my pistol is a tool used to fight my way to my rifle. Police officers keep a rifle in their trunk and don't typically take them out on calls with them but instead retrieve them reactively. This practice is tailored to law enforcement, who have a much greater chance of encountering danger than a normal civilian. Keeping a rifle ready to go in your home is a perfectly acceptable practice and can arguably be used as a staging point to fight with your pistol.

I love the idea of a get-home bag. A get-home bag is something that is thrown in your trunk and deployed in an extreme situation where it is tactically reasonable to abandon your vehicle and use the bag to get home. While I understand this sounds like a crazy notion, imagine getting stuck in a flood, wildfire, or even a civil disturbance where you are trapped. Don't worry, I'm sure insurance will cover it. Grab your get-home bag and begin your trek to safety. Much like keeping a rifle as a fundamental EDC tool, I don't foresee myself taking a get-home bag to the mailbox with me, and for this reason, I don't have it on my essentials list.

Finally, food and water supplies are not on my essentials list simply because I think of it as a supply more than an EDC tool. Many tactical gurus suggest that EDC with a water bladder or an MRE is a good habit to form. I, however, can't entirely agree due to the simple fact that you will not always carry an MRE and a Camelback every day. Remember, EDC and survival are two different things, even though they have many similarities and can be easily mistaken for one another.

One more important note: EDC is something that takes time to perfect. If you are not used to carrying gear besides a wallet and phone, it will probably feel foreign at first. If you start carrying a pistol, you will often be hyper-focused on it in public. Try not to think about it too much. This could lead to compulsively touching your hip to feel that it's in place, giving away to everyone around you (who knows what they're looking at) that you are armed. Ensure that you have a good holster, and it will not go anywhere. Make sure your gear is comfortable. Having uncomfortable gear is one of the biggest reasons why people don't carry it, and EDC is every single day. The more you carry it, the more normal it will become. This includes your firearm, a knife, a flashlight, and whatever else you determine to be essential to carry daily.

Also, something to think about is the clothing you choose to wear. I like the phrase "Dress around your gun." In my opinion, my firearm is the most cumbersome piece of tactical gear that I carry. It's the largest and the hardest to conceal. Dressing around my gun means that I plan to wear my gun before I choose what clothing I'm going to wear. This means that if I carry a larger gun, I will not wear gym shorts and a tight shirt. If I'm planning to have a micro-compact pistol, I can probably get away with a pocket holster that will conceal it just fine in shorts. I have the luxury of owning different carry options, but if you are looking for an all-purpose EDC carry gun, consider that before you choose one.

Danger/ Target Zones to Avoid

In the spirit of confrontation elusion, several places should be avoided to maximize your chances of safety and tactical superiority. These places are by no means a total no-go but generally offer less security than other locations. Consider these geographical locations to be one step higher on your risk assessment. Of course, it goes without saying that no place is completely off limits, but the places I speak about below are places where an attack is more likely to occur and deserve a higher-level of attentiveness.

Gun Free Zones

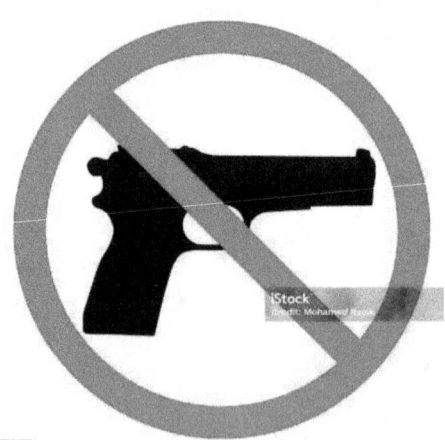

First on this list is no gun zones. These areas (commonly businesses or private property establishments) post signs that advise against carrying concealed weapons. To state the obvious, this puts you at a disadvantage because it is down grading your personal defense options should a dangerous situation arise. I regularly ignore these zones due to the illegal signage or the simple fact that I believe in the Second Amendment, but do your research into local and state laws and make an educated decision. No gun zones also provide insight and even a potential target for criminals to take advantage of. As I've said before, criminals are opportunists and would much rather exploit a place where they believe everyone is unarmed than a place where they may have to enter a gun fight.

Bars & Night Clubs

Next on the list are bars and night clubs. As an adult with traditional values and an old soul, I don't find these places as appealing as they were when I was 21. However, I am aware that patriots come in all ages, and this needs to be on the list. Night clubs and bars typically have multiple elements that can escalate danger. There is alcohol, which lessens the ability to make a sound decision, lowers reaction speed, and (in the state of South Carolina) makes it illegal to have a firearm on your person during consumption. Also, these establishments commonly attract young male and female patrons and are used as a hub for romantic networking. Putting the equation together, we have young men trying to pick up a lady, alcohol all around, making people unreasonable, and a lack of legal firearms. Sounds like a good spot to add to the "no-fly" list, in my opinion. The best option you have if you find yourself in a bar or nightclub is not to overindulge and stay alert to escalating situations around you.

Heavily Populated Areas

Heavily populated areas are next on this list. I understand this is a vague statement, but it's by design. One of the elements of an active shooter situation is a target-rich environment. If we think about where that normally is (a church, a concert, a night club, a school), we will have a good illustration that this is a true statement. I always think of a large crowd of people as a risk and avoid it if there is another option. Understandably, people do have a social life, and often, this includes going to events with friends. Add this to your risk assessment and make a right decision for you.

Wide Open Spaces

Finally, I tend to avoid wide open spaces. When I was in basic training for the army, we had an area in our barracks called the 'kill zone'. This area was in the center of the room and had a different color painted on the floor. This area was *never* to be walked on and was meticulously maintained by the fireguard shift every night after lights out. We polished this zone until it was as reflective as a car. We could avoid this zone even if we were sleepwalking because it was so ingrained in our psyche to do so.

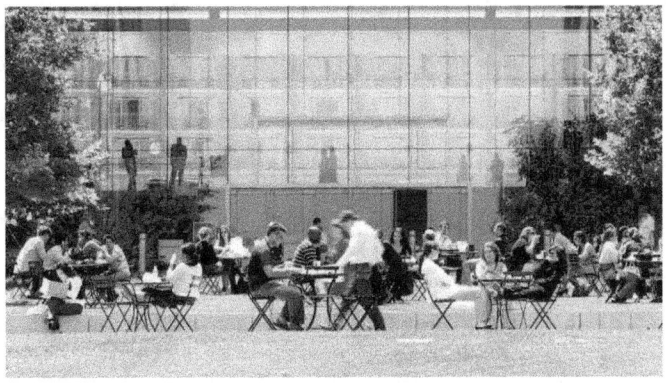

For the longest time, I didn't understand why this zone was part of the rules, but I did what I was told and continued avoiding it. Fast forward to my law enforcement career, when I started regularly becoming involved in specialized teams, tactical entry situations, and CQB, I realized the kill zone was all too real. The kill zone was the center of the room, where you could be seen from all angles. The place where there was the least amount of cover and concealment. It was the place where you were most likely to be killed. I apply this principal to exterior geographical areas as well. I tend to avoid areas that have no usable cover, if possible. This includes places like empty parking lots, concert audience fields, and even when I choose my seat in church. Stick to the outside and survive.

Proper Training

As a former training supervisor for the State of South Carolina, this topic is near and dear to my heart. Training could possibly be the most important topic in this entire book. When training others, I always attempted to follow the guide of cognitive, affective, and psychomotor training. Simply put, this means tell me, show me, and let me try it. This format has been proven throughout decades of training with thousands of law enforcement and military agencies. Typically, this training style comes in the form of a PowerPoint presentation, followed by a demonstration by the instructor(s), and finally, a hands-on portion where you get to try it out yourself.

However, from the perspective of a civilian who is trying to self-train, this can be difficult. Having a training partner when doing physical training is always encouraged, but the first two portions can simply be done without one. Should you research a topic online, you will find that there are millions of resources that can be used to teach you a technique and demonstrate it for you. It is also important to understand *Hicks Law*. To summarize, Hicks Law states that the more information you are given, the less information you will retain. This means that if you try to learn too much at one time, you will ultimately learn less than you would if you focused on a smaller portion of the training. For example, instead of learning 100 words a day in Spanish, you will find more value if you try to learn 10 words daily. This will allow you to concentrate on each word more, giving you less information to comprehend and making it easier to retain.

Before transitioning into different types of training, it's important to identify different levels of training intensity and which one is appropriate for your current situation and skill level. Bear in mind, these are just guidelines, and your training can be flexible in either direction.

Academic Training (Theory)

Academic Training is the "classroom" portion of your training. This step is where you learn what it is you will be practicing, how to do it properly, and why this method is superior. This is the "tell me" Portion of your training.

Static Training

Static training is the starting level of physical training. This is typically where the "show me" portion of your training comes in. Static training usually breaks down each individual movement and goes through step by step. For example, if you are learning how to make a peanut butter sandwich, static training will show the instructor how to scoop the peanut butter out of the jar with a knife and then spread it onto the bread before checking for understanding. Each step is described in detail as the instructor shows you.

Fluid Training

Fluid training is the first step in putting theory into practice. This is where you begin the "let me do it" phase of training and advance through the various steps in slow motion. Fluid training is designed to get your body used to the different motions that you will eventually do quickly. Think about when you see a golfer line up to take a shot. Often, they will step to the side and take a few practice swings that are slower than normal but essentially use the same movements. This is a good example of fluid training. You're going through the motions to get used to them before taking the swing for real.

Dynamic Training

Dynamic training is where you put all the steps together and try it for real. This of this training as an attempt at a maximum bench press. This type of training gives you the best understanding and the most valuable practice. However, it puts you at the highest risk for injury as well. Dynamic training typically doesn't go over 80% effort. This is by design and leaves a cushion in the hopes that you don't push beyond your capabilities and get hurt. Dynamic training is often seen in martial arts gyms for live sparring or in combat sports for exhibition matches. While I do see the benefit in dynamic training, I do not recommend this as a regular form of training, as the risk of injury is much higher than seen in fluid training.

As previously stated, training levels can be shifted up or down depending on training needs. For example, you can spend most of your time doing fluid training to learn a new technique and get comfortable with the movements before transitioning to a short dynamic training at the end to reenforce the learning. This is a common practice in most martial arts gyms and sports practices, as it gives you a lot of bang for your buck.

Finally, it should be noted that training is required for everything. Whether it's eating with a fork or performing brain surgery, there is always some level of training required to do it properly. This training philosophy should open your eyes to your strengths and weaknesses in all tactical aspects of your life. Have you been trained in risk management? Have you trained and practiced dynamic driving in your vehicle? Do you know how to draw your firearm while sitting down properly? Small things like these that you don't necessarily think about could mean the difference between life and death in a dangerous situation.

"Fire Drills"

You learned it in school and never thought anything of it. The fire alarm sounds, and everyone calmly gets up and into a single file line before leaving the building through the nearest exit. If you can remember, you never got scared during these drills, and they weren't usually a big deal. This is because of the number of drills that occurred throughout your grade school years. You may have been excited for the first one and maybe the second, but by the time you were in high school, this was just a minor inconvenience to your day.

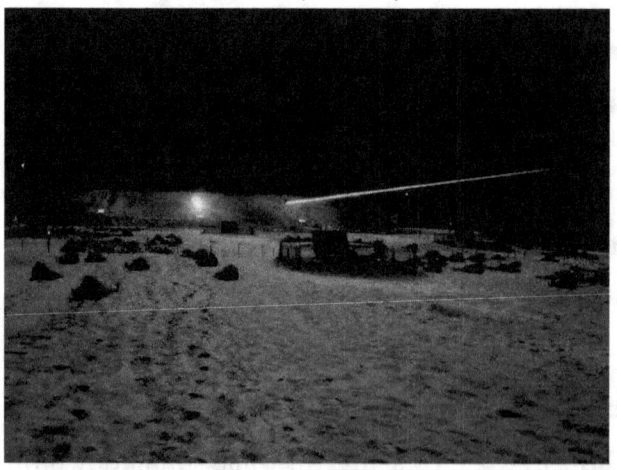

Desensitizing yourself to danger is one of the best ways to control it. In the military, we conducted a training called NIC at Night. During this training, we were tasked to crawl across a 100-yard field in the dark while our instructors shot 50 caliber tracer rounds over our heads from an M2 machine gun. The entire purpose of this training was to give us the experience of reacting to gunfire, desensitizing us to it.

Now, put theory into practice, and you'll start to wonder why we don't use danger drills at home. Why do we not teach our children how to react to a fire at our house? Why don't we have home invasion drills? Why don't we practice leaving our home and rapidly deploying our vehicle with the whole family? These drills may seem ridiculous, but the harsh reality is that these are the movements you will be forced to conduct if a dangerous situation occurs. There should be a safe zone in your home that your family can go to should there be a home invasion. This space should have a secondary means of escape, some concealment from the rest of the house, and a weapon (preferably a firearm) stagged there for a last-stand defense. It may sound paranoid, but so did seat belts when they were first invented.

Danger Drills are an effective way to react effectively in a chaotic situation. By using repetition and desensitization to an incident that normally creates terror or panic, you and your family can have the upper hand and be prepared for just about anything. While I'm not necessarily encouraging you to be a doomsday prepper, I am promoting a general residential preparedness for common threats and risks. You have a car with seatbelts to prepare for collisions, you have a fire extinguisher to prepare for a fire in your home, and you have locks on your doors to keep out unwanted people. You have all these protections in place, so why wouldn't you have other protections for other dangerous situations? As with everything we talk about in this book, danger drills should be specific to your area. If you are in Florida, you should not practice reacting to an avalanche. If you live on the side of a mountain at the end of a private road, drive-by shootings shouldn't be on your list of things to prepare for. Sit down with your family and review a normal day. Make a list of common actions and a list of common threats. Prioritize what is the biggest threat and begin a rotation that goes down the list. Even practicing once per month can set your family up for success in the presence of danger.

Ethics vs. Morals

Ethics vs. Morals is a timeless debate about the fundamental differences between right and wrong. When you think about being dangerous and ensuring safety for yourself and your loved ones, ethics and morals are often overlooked. A classic example of ethics vs. morals is the scenario of "Would you steal bread to feed your starving family." Every state in the nation has a law against theft. Theft is even written in the 10 commandments as being wrong.

As humans, we subconsciously assign value to everything. If you're a person who values family above all else, you would probably steal the bread despite it being a breach of ethics. Ultimately, you decide that you would not be able to look yourself in the mirror if you allowed your family to starve, knowing there was something you could do about it. Morally, you had to help your family, although ethically, you knew it was wrong.

This same conversation can be had when you are thinking about proactive self-defense. Many state laws support a "stand your ground" clause or a "Castle Doctrine." This states that there is no expectation to flee from a deadly threat and that force up to lethal force can be used to protect yourself or others. In the debate of ethics vs. morals, however, you must be able to make the conscientious decision to act or to flee. I am a patriot to my core, and I value the Constitution above many aspects of my life. I understand what it means to take a life, and I also understand the potential consequences of that action. Do you value your material things over another human life? Can you be the one who can live with yourself after taking another's life? What if you did it to defend your family from a lethal threat? Ultimately, this decision-making process can get you killed. If I am faced with a threat and I am with my family, I must be prepared to make a life-changing decision and shouldn't hesitate to debate myself in the heat of the moment.

Much like danger drills, this is a topic that you can train to desensitize yourself to. To accomplish this, have conversations with trusted family friends about what would happen in dangerous situations. This can easily happen by watching movies with loved ones. Often, I'll watch a crime movie with my wife and see a dangerous incident occur. I'll talk with her about it and say something like, "Just so you know, if this ever happens to us, I would …" This is a great way to get these conversions started without looking like a paranoid lunatic.

Is The Juice Worth the Squeeze?

Within any aspect of tactics, there is a balance, a give and take that allows you to make decisions that will ultimately determine the outcome of any given situation. When making decisions, especially in a dynamic situation, you must choose whether sacrifices that are being made add value to the goal or mission. *Is the juice worth the squeeze?* An active shooter incident can illustrate a basic example of this.

Picture this: you're at a local restaurant eating lunch alone. There is a decent-sized crowd in the business, and you have made the proper risk assessments and are positioned in the back near an exit. Suddenly, someone comes through the front door and starts shooting in the air, screaming that they are robbing everyone. You are armed and have a clear shot at the target with no one behind them. Do you take out your gun and shoot? Often, when given this scenario, a dangerous person would say yes. They would take out their gun and shoot the criminals, saving themselves and potentially saving the lives of everyone else in the establishment. Understand that by taking out your gun, you have ultimately made yourself the largest target in the room to the criminal. Should you miss, should your gun malfunction, should the criminal see you drawing your weapon and happen to be faster, you are dead. Even under these circumstances, a dangerous person would typically agree that they would still attempt to fire upon the criminal.

Now, picture the same scenario. However, you are with your children, best friends, and loved ones. Does your action plan change? Now, you must decide if the juice is worth the squeeze. When it was just your safety on the line, the decision was rather easy, but now you have the safety of your loved ones to consider as well. Many times, when presented with this version of the scenario, the action plan changes, and the dangerous person will choose to protect the retreat of their loved ones as they exit the building. Often, they have decided that the juice wasn't worth the squeeze.

This isn't a scenario that has a right and wrong answer, but instead is designed to make you think about how your actions have reactions, and help you determine value and importance to your situation. If I find myself on a date with my wife and there is a life-threatening situation that occurs, my main plan of action is to get my wife to safety. This may be controversial, but it is honest. Mentally preparing yourself for these decisions early on will help you respond more efficiently to the situation when confronted with it. Play the "what if" game early and often and begin the process of desensitizing yourself to these decisions. When it's planned, it will be much easier to accomplish.

To take it a step further, consider larger-scale decisions you make in your life and apply this question. Should I leave this steady 9-5 job for a riskier role with larger earning potential? Should I go back to school even though I'm in my mid 40's? Despite the danger, should I go skydiving like I've always wanted to? Analyze the risk, decide based on value vs. threat of loss, and add variables at the end. What do I have to gain if I leave my 9-5 for a risky business venture? Potentially making a million dollars in a year. What is the threat of loss? The plan doesn't work out and now I'm unemployed, with no steady income stream. Now add variables: are you independent and providing for only yourself? Do you own valuable assets that could be lost from this risk, and how soon can you acquire another 9-5 position? The point of this assessment is to be able to use it fluidly. You can create plans for vacations with your family. You can create your "fire drills" based on this assessment. You can use this tool to determine your long-term goals and milestones. It's a universal assessment tool that can be used to be dangerous or to avoid danger.

Observe, Orient, Decide, Act

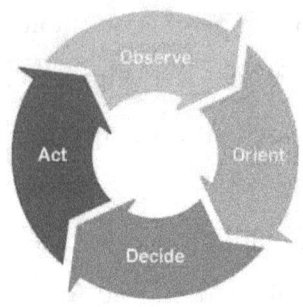

Observe, Orient, Decide, and Act (OODA), often referred to as the 'OODA Loop', is a psychological theory first created by U.S. Air Force Colonel John Boyd and was created to help conceptualize combat cognitive processes during dynamic military situations. This philosophy explains the human's psychological process when tasked with a decision. This process starts with observing a threat by seeing it physically in front of you. In the next phase, you orient that it is indeed a threat to you, identifying it as dangerous and preparing yourself to decide. Next, you decide to either engage that threat or flee. Finally, you act on your decision, physically taking the step you decided on. This is the entire cognitive process a person goes through for every decision.

To put it to a normal, real-world perspective, think of observing an object instead of observing a threat. For example, driving down the road, you see a traffic light. You observe that there is a traffic light that is showing green because you see it in front of you. You orient that the light is illuminating green, which signals you to go and prepare your mind to decide what to do. You decide to continue driving through the light and act upon that decision by doing it. A real-world scenario that most people will encounter daily.

Now, the OODA Loop theory can be dangerous when we encounter the "Loop" part. The loop is included because should the OODA process be interrupted at any point, the brain must restart the process. It may not seem that way because this process happens so quickly, but it's true. Once the OODA is interrupted, you must start over. Commonly, you will find that the OODA process is interrupted by introducing another choice. Another object to observe has entered the situation, disturbing you and stopping you from deciding and acting upon it. In a military setting, this could be a soldier who is about to engage an enemy combatant with their rifle when, just before they pull the trigger, a second threat enters the area. Now, the person is faced with another OODA process they must do before they have completed the first one. This becomes a dangerous situation because it causes hesitation, which takes up valuable time.

Still don't believe me? Let's put this situation back into a real-world setting. Let's imagine the traffic light again: You're driving down the road and approaching a traffic light. You observe that there is a traffic light, orient that the light is green as you approach the intersection, and decide that you're going to travel through the light. Now, just before you act, the light turns yellow, and suddenly, your foot starts to dance back and forth between the gas and the break, and you stop a little bit before ultimately running the now red light. You were caught in the OODA Loop. Your process was interrupted by an introduction of a secondary factor, causing you to hesitate. While it may not be a big deal in the traffic light situation, this can play a huge role in a combat situation. So, how do you fight your mind's natural cognitive process and beat the OODA Loop? To be candid, you can't. However, you can take steps to minimize the impact it has on you and your actions in a dangerous situation.

Understand Your Mind

First, understanding the OODA Loop and how your mind works will make you more aware of your experiences. If I know that I have a food allergy, I am going to be much more aware of the foods that I put in my body. I haven't changed my biology; I still need to eat. Instead, I added a factor to help me prepare for a bad situation. I learned about OODA and how it can cause hesitation, and I began to recognize it more often as it's happening in everyday situations.

Practice Deciding and Acting Simultaneously

Before you start trying to decide and act simultaneously, understand that it is impossible. The purpose of this exercise is to train yourself to make decisions quickly. For example, I know that I can't breathe in and out simultaneously; it's impossible. However, if I asked you to try it, you would undoubtedly breathe in once and breathe out once very rapidly. I never said to do it quickly in my instructions, but it's my mind's natural response to try to trick myself with surprise. Use this in your training and when you find yourself hesitating, make a quick decision and stick to it, even though you have your split-second doubts. If you do this enough, you'll develop a quick decision-making pattern that helps you break the loop.

Understand that this concept is not a one-size-fits-all and should be used as just one of the many tools in your tool belt. The OODA Loop is not going anywhere, but like everything else discussed in this book, training and practice will prepare you for real and dangerous incidents.

Risk Mitigation

So, we have now determined that we are easy to kill and why. We know that the odds are stacked against us, and we will more than likely be targeted due to our inexperience and failure to develop our abilities proactively. Luckily, there are steps you can take right now that will instantly make you safer and less likely to be a victim.

Situational Awareness

The next time you go into a public place, take a second and look around. Chances are that you will see people with their heads down looking at their phones. This could be at a sporting event, a bar, a restaurant, a concert, or anywhere else where people congregate. Media distraction is dangerous. People live second lives on social media and often spend as much time on their phones as they do asleep at night, if not more. While it isn't a sexy subject, situational awareness is arguably one of the most important elements of a dangerous person. Being aware of your surroundings and identifying risks could help you avoid confrontation, stop a sucker punch, or even save yourself and your loved ones from a rampage killer.

Just break down the phrase (Situation/ Aware) to be situationally aware. What situation are you in right now? Maybe you're sitting on your couch with a cup of tea, reading this book in the peace and quiet of your home. Maybe you're on the subway, reading this book to take your mind off the creepy guy who keeps staring at you from the other end of the rail car. Maybe you're in a coffee shop enjoying a dark roast on your day off. Three different scenarios, all with the potential to be a victim.

You're at home and relaxing on your couch, and you don't see the headlights pass your windows as a car pulls into your driveway. You're enjoying the book so much that you may not hear the window break on the other side of the house. Maybe you have a little music on, and it blocks the sound of footsteps coming down the hall. You have just become a victim. You're on the subway reading a book. You notice the creepy guy looking at you but pay him no attention (you don't want to judge a book by its cover, right?). You politely ignore the obviously inappropriate glaring and mind your own business, not realizing that he is texting your description to a human trafficker on the next car down. You exit the train feeling relief that the creepy guy was left behind and "safely" begin your walk home. You have just become a victim. You're sitting in a coffee shop relaxing on your day off. You're sipping your delicious coffee and not paying attention to the room around you, failing to see the person crying at the other end while being fired from his job. He reaches into his pocket for the cold steel he uses to take out as many people as he can before ending his life. You have just become a victim.

Sure, you can tell yourself that these situations are extreme and likely won't happen to you. You're right, they probably won't. However, these situations have happened and continue to happen in every state nationwide. At the end of the day, no matter what your religion, political preference, race, or social status, you can still become a victim. The people who train for these situations, prepare for the worst, hope for the best, and continuously conduct risk assessments are the ones who will be more likely to survive.

Enter a room and look for the exits. Make a mental note of where they are and how close you are to them. Many public establishments will have a fire evacuation plan that is posted close to the entrance of the building. This plan can show you all the exits and give you more information about the layout of the building that may be helpful in a dynamic situation.

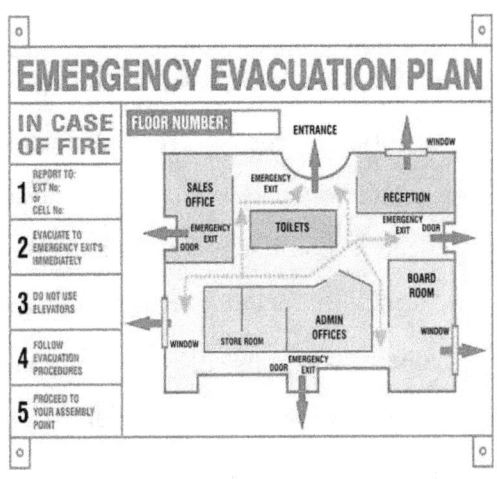

The best way to win in a violent situation is to exclude yourself from it. If you are close to an exit and can remove yourself from the equation, do it. Being close to an exit gives you the option to leave, which can prove to be invaluable in a life-and-death situation. However, making a quick escape isn't always possible, so don't count on it as your only option.

Look at the people in the room and find the biggest threat. This can be difficult because truly dangerous people will not always stand out but instead blend with their surroundings (much like the ambush predators we mentioned earlier). Look at their body language. Look for someone who doesn't like to have their back to the door or prefers to stay outside the room with their back against the wall. Look for visual clues on the attire of the threat. Signs of military experience include flags, wearing combat boots or hats, or having military tattoos. Signs of gang activity can be very similar to military personnel. Physical fitness and body signs are great indicators of danger. If someone has a cauliflower ear, it can be assumed that they are very experienced in combat sports. If someone has visual scars or callused knuckles, this may suggest they are a fighter.

Identify potential weapons of opportunity. There are thousands of educational resources on identifying and using weapons of opportunity. However, the element that is commonly missed is putting practice into action. You see it in movies all the time: the star gets into this 5-minute fistfight with the bad guy and hits him with bottles, lamps, pool cues, chairs, and anything else they can get their hands on. The reality is that fights do not happen this way. If someone smashes a liquor bottle over your head, you will be knocked unconscious and may even die from the experience. Blunt-force trauma is rarely represented accurately in movies, giving us an unrealistic perspective of violent confrontations. People don't get knocked out every time they get punched in the face. Having an unrealistic idea of what happens in combat can be a weakness in battle.

<u>*Blending In*</u>

Blending in with an environment is a tool that is used by some of the most dangerous people on earth. Often referred to as 'The Grey Man Theory', this method is used to disappear into a crowd and effectively maneuver otherwise challenging obstacles. If you picture an assassin, what comes to mind? Do you see a person dressed like a ninja, with a face shroud and a sniper rifle, engaging a threat from afar? Do you imagine a James Bond-style agent dressed in a tuxedo and armed with a toxic poison and a suppressed pistol? Factually, assassins and professional killers don't get caught because they don't stand out. If you were at a fancy dinner party where everyone is dressed in a suit, and an assailant kicks down the door wearing a camo jumpsuit, face paint, a bandolier of bullets and holding a machine gun, you would immediately know that person was a threat. The element of surprise comes with the value that no one knows your intentions, capabilities, or skills and experience.

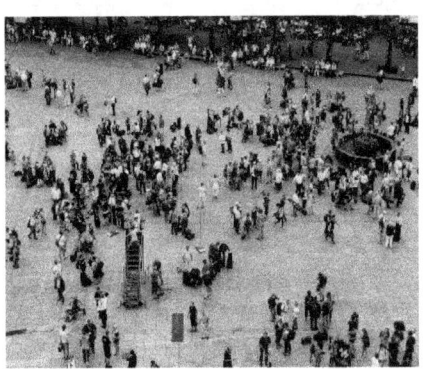

Blending in with modern society can be something as little as wearing flip-flops. Have you ever seen a movie where a murderer runs around in flip-flops? How about the action hero, beating his way through a street gang in jean shorts? While I'm not advising you to dress like a middle-aged father in Florida, I suggest that wearing unsuspecting clothing can be as valuable to you as having a weapon. If you are a military veteran, maybe consider leaving the multi-cam clothes in the closet. Combat boots look cool but aren't necessary in the civilian world. No one is impressed with your dog tags (sorry). If you have a concealed weapons permit, ensure your weapon is completely concealed, and don't tell people about it (even though you think it looks super-cool to open carry it).

Tactical Positioning

As mentioned above, many people refuse to sit with their backs to the door. Some refer to it as a cowboy function, and others see it as general paranoia or PTSD. Many people who take this position will never get value from it and don't know how to maximize the safety that comes with it. There are other factors besides being able to see the door that you should consider when deciding your positioning in a public setting. The first thing to do is think about tactical priority.

Tactical priority means you assess what is the most immediate danger to you in this public setting and what threats may be less immediate. Giving more threatening elements priority over others can give you the advantage if a violent situation occurs. For example, I enter a restaurant with my date, and I see a man sitting in the middle of the room with a firearm on his hip. He doesn't appear to be law enforcement and has no one else with him. I note that the door I came through is the only accessible exit in the room. Also, an elderly couple is sitting towards the back of the room by the restrooms. I will choose to sit so I can have a clear route to the exit while also maintaining a clear visual of the man with the gun. This may entail having my back to the elderly couple sitting in the booth behind me, but that is a much lesser risk than a man with a gun. I prioritize the armed civilian, followed by the unknown threat of the doorway and only potential exit, and finally, the elderly couple.

A final consideration of your positioning is whether you are trapped in a space. This means that there is a threat between you and the doorway. Some may argue that this is "Stacking the threats." However, in a civilian society, exiting a violent confrontation should always be the first response (if possible). I would much rather triangulate the threat with the door, leaving me a clear escape route instead of forcing me to go through the threat to retreat.

Reticular Activating System (RAS)

A great tool to use passively while maintaining situational awareness is your Reticular Activating System (RAS). The RAS is a group of nerves located at the bottom of the brainstem and functions by controlling consciousness and demeanor. In other words, it takes in information from your brain and decides how you'll react to that information.

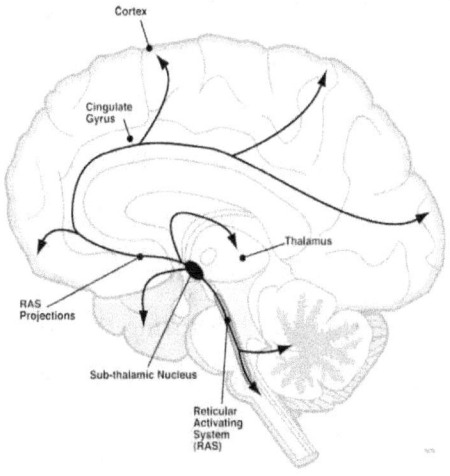

Often, people use the example of buying a unique car. If I go to the car dealership and decide that I want to buy a car because it's in a new exclusive color (say orange, for example). I've never seen that color on a car before, and the chances are that someone else somewhere has purchased this car in this color for the same reason. However, once you buy it and start to drive it around, you'll notice that there are already a lot of the same cars in that color already on the road. How can this be? Earlier that same day, when you drove to the dealership, you were certain that you'd never seen that combination before, and now it's everywhere. Your RAS has engaged for this specific combination and told you to react because it's distinctive and unique.

So, how is this relevant to becoming dangerous? The RAS exists to keep you alive by automation. This means the brain makes identifications and reactions based on what we identify as requiring attention. A good example of this is a person in the military. It is not uncommon for deployed soldiers to react automatically to certain things once they get home. For example, if a car tire blows out on the road nearby, it may sound like a gunshot or bomb, causing the soldier to drop to the ground or take cover. This isn't caused by PTSD (though it may trigger an episode), but in fact, it is caused by the RAS telling you to alert and react to that certain sound.

We have covered the information on risk assessments and situational awareness. We know that there are certain things that we should look for that would cause a tactical "red flag" if we see it. We can train ourselves to use the RAS to our advantage by spending time looking for these important indicators and threats and identifying them. We can watch people in the mall or Walmart as they grab the gun in the front of their pants and adjust it. We can watch for people in restaurants who refuse to sit with their back to the room. We can smell the odor of narcotics on people as they drive past or walk near us. We can see the pocket clip of the knife in someone's jeans.

Once we spend enough time looking for and identifying these types of threats, your RAS will determine that it's important and you will begin to do it automatically. If you are a prior law enforcement officer, you will automatically look at the violations on vehicles as you drive down the interstate. If you're a chef, you'll constantly be looking at the cleanliness of any other food establishment you go to. If you are a writer, you'll be more inclined to catch grammar errors in a book or magazine. Repetition is the key to programming automation in your body. Once your RAS has identified these indicators, you will have no choice but to be more aware of your surroundings.

Even more impressive than that is the ability to use the RAS as an automation tool in your everyday life actions. If you choose to hyper-focus on certain things throughout the day that are required for your safety, you will eventually begin to do them automatically. A good example is driving. Have you ever been driving home after a long day at work or traveling on a long trip and forget that you are driving? Maybe you have traveled a mile or two and realized you don't remember any of it. You weren't daydreaming, but it was like you were on autopilot. Your RAS took over as you did not have the cognitive ability at that moment to act. So, instead of automating dangerous things like driving, focus on locking your front door any time you walk through it. Focus on the exact placement of your EDC firearm and how it would feel to draw from your different positions throughout the day. Focus on going straight to the gym after work as if it's a part of your day every day. Eventually, this will become automatic and make you much more efficient.

The Fundamentals of Marksmanship

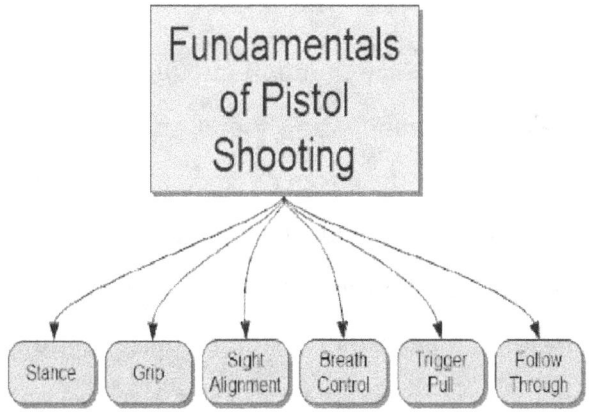

This chapter is not going to be what you think it is. As a firearms instructor, a US Army veteran, a former SRT Commander, and a firearms enthusiast, it has been ingrained in me that the fundamentals of marksmanship are the most important elements of good shooting. To a point, I agree, but there are some exceptions as well. If you are a long-distance precision marksman, you absolutely need to think about every one of the fundamentals of Marksmanship. If you are a competitive shooter for long guns or pistols, you must use the fundamentals to ensure peak performance. However, if you are not focused on the competition, hitting a target at 1000 yards, or shooting steel under a timer, I would argue that the fundamentals of marksmanship are not the most important things. Stick with me.

Stance

Stance on a gun range is important. One of the things that tilts the scales between a good shooter and a great shooter is repeatability. Having the proper stance allows you comfort, stability, control, and the ability to shoot repeatedly while being accurate. However, in a self-defense situation, stance is more than likely not in the equation. More than likely, you will be in a confrontation of sorts. Sit in a car or chair or stand close quarters with someone as you fight for your life. Maybe you're attempting to get away while someone pursues you with the intention of doing you harm. It is not reasonable to worry about proper stance in this situation. For this reason, I typically don't recommend training in a gun range while shooting at paper. The chances are that you are going to be on the move when firing your weapon.

Sight Alignment

Sight alignment is another very important element to remember while you are shooting at the gun range. To be able to shoot to the accuracy capability of your firearm, you need to ensure that your front sight and rear sights are properly aligned. This statement is true for both pistols and rifles alike.

However, in self-defense, people often don't even use their sight. I understand how ridiculous that sounds, but I promise it's true. In fact, many law enforcement, military, and private contractors conduct CQB training with only their front sights to reinforce their movement patterns. This is because most gun fights occur within a few feet. A good rule of thumb is if you can confidently point a finger at a particular spot on someone's body, you can shoot it.

Sight Picture

A proper sight picture can be the difference between a hit and a missed shot at a distance. Again, falling back to the same argument we saw above, most people involved in a gunfight won't use sights at all. Understand that I do not agree with shooting with no sights, but that is realistically what happens. For someone who is a beginner who wants to stay safe while being able to defend themselves, there are more important things to focus on.

Proper Grip

This is a good one to focus on. Ensuring you have a proper grip on your gun can and will certainly change how you perform, especially under pressure. Know that your grip starts while the gun is still in the holster. When you practice shooting, you do not have the proper grip if you constantly adjust your hands between rounds. There are many different methods of gripping a handgun, many of which are terrible. Understand that your gun has texture on the grip for a reason. When shooting, your hands fill as much of that real estate as possible. The heel of both of your palms should be in contact with the texturized grip of your gun. Your fingers should be aligned with each other, with your weak hand on top of your strong hand. If done properly, both of your thumbs should point forward while aligning with the gun's rail. Ensure that the webbing of your hand between the thumb and pointer finger on the strong hand is choked up as far as it can go to the slide. Most guns, such as Glock or S&W and all 1911-style pistols, have a beaver tail (or a variation of one) to stop your hand from getting bitten by the slide cycling. Slide bite occurs when you are gripping the gun improperly. When you draw your weapon from the holster, you should grab it with your hand already choked up as far as it will go. This will create more space for your support hand and make your drawing faster and more accurate.

Breathing

Breathing is arguably important for self-defense but not for the sake of marksmanship. I truly believe in combat meditation, tactical breathing, and using breathing methods to break tunnel vision and maintain awareness. The fundamentals of marksmanship focus on maintaining controlled breaths so they do not move your sight picture or create an unstable platform while shooting. This is obviously a moot point when you're fighting for your life or shooting in self-defense.

Trigger Control

This one is going to be short and sweet. Trigger control is both important and not important. I say this because I think of trigger control as keeping your finger out of the trigger guard until you're ready to shoot something. The safety side of this is a green light. Even in a firefight while running and gunning, you will not find my finger inside the trigger guard when I'm not shooting. It takes practice, but it is certainly possible. Trigger squeeze is what the fundamentals of marksmanship refer to, and it doesn't matter in self-defense. You will not slowly squeeze the trigger until the gun discharges. You will not use the trigger reset by feeling a bump and hearing a metallic click. It would be great if you did, but you won't. In self-defense, the only thing you will be able to focus on is the person who's trying to kill you. For the same reason, you won't use your sights. You won't use proper trigger squeeze.

Follow Through

Follow-through is important not only because it makes you more accurate but also because it keeps you in the fight. Many trainers will have students "scan for threats" before holstering their weapons. This isn't because they believe the boogeyman is going to pop out and surprise them, but more realistically, it will help break tunnel vision and keep you aware of your surroundings. For example, if you get into a shooting and put rounds into someone, you are going to be locked into that person visually. By training to scan after shooting, you are training to break the tunnel vision and look around you. You may find that after a shooting, you are standing in the middle of the street, or there is another bad guy next to you, or even more likely, there are law enforcement officers approaching who don't know what's going on. Being able to analyze the situation quickly is important because the moments after a self-defense shooting are almost as dangerous as the shooting itself.

Quick and Easy Skills and Tactics

Remembering the difference between skills and tactics, we can now talk about quick and easy drills you can use to continue your tactical development. For the sake of simplicity, and since this is a beginner manual, I will keep this chapter focused on the use of firearms. Understand, however, that skills and tactics exist for any tool or practice, and I encourage you to branch out and seek more understanding for the tools you will be relying on every day.

<u>Skills</u>

1. Magazine Changes

Empty your firearm. Empty all your magazines. Ensure they are all empty and there is no ammunition in the area at all. Now, take your firearm to the bedroom and stand over your bed. Draw your firearm from the holster and point it as if you're engaging a target. Drop your magazine to the ground (bed) and reload another magazine before again pointing the gun as if you're engaging a target. Repeat. This seems simple because it is. Doing this easy drill is a way to establish muscle memory and become faster at reloading under pressure.

2. Dry Firing

Empty your firearm. Empty your magazine. Ensure they are both empty and there is no ammunition in the area at all. Now, rack the slide on your firearm so that the pistol is cocked and ready to fire. Point the gun in a safe direction and slowly pull the trigger until the gun is 'fired'. Hold the trigger back while you again rack the slide to cock the gun. Slowly release the trigger until you feel/ hear a metallic click. That is your trigger reset. Once you feel that, pull the trigger again. Repeat. This process is called dry fire. It's a method used to practice proper trigger squeeze and trigger reset. I do this constantly. I do it while watching TV, I do it while I'm relaxing around the house, and I do this whenever I have free time. The more you do this, the better your trigger squeeze will be. Note: if you're going to do this with a rim fire pistol or a revolver, it is recommended that you get "snap caps" or dud rounds to practice with to avoid damaging your firearm.

3. Transitions

You can do this drill while at the range or home. This is completed by successfully transitioning from a rifle to a pistol. We transition like this anytime you're actively engaging a target and encounter a jam or when you run out of ammunition. Instead of wasting time under fire to clear a jam and/or reload, transition to your sidearm, and stay in the fight. This is accomplished by first having your rifle at the ready as if you're engaging a target. While your rifle has a sling on it, lower it to the side of your body, opposite your dominant side. For example, the rifle will go to your left side if you are right-handed. Once lowered, retrieve your sidearm from the holster and present it to engage a target. As you complete this drill, focus on lowering the rifle while simultaneously drawing the pistol. This movement should almost be fluid, completing both movements only moments apart.

4. Reflexive Fire

Reflexive fire is done at the range with a partner. Get a target with multiple shapes with numbers inside them (the fancy ones are even different colors). These can be bought or made. Either one is fine. Now, from the holster, have your range buddy call out a shape, a number, or a color, and you engage what he calls. A simple concept but can prove difficult as you progress through the drill. Once you get the hang of it, have your buddy call different options simultaneously, i.e., "Yellow, Triangle, Two" and you have to engage all that apply. This drill teaches you to establish your operational speed while making you quicker with practice.

5. Incapacitation Drills (Jam Clearing)

This one is always fun. This drill is done with a buddy. Have a buddy load a magazine for your gun and add a blank somewhere randomly inside. While you are shooting and engaging targets, you will inevitably encounter a blank or "malfunction" completely incapacitating your round of fire. You must clear the jam as quickly as possible and get back into the fight. These jams can be added multiple times or combined with other drills, such as reflexive fire, to maximize training value. Please note that this is typically not an authorized drill at public ranges. Consult the range safety officer or ensure you are at a safe and private range prior to attempting this drill.

6. Weapon Retention

This drill is more of a combat drill; however, it is very straightforward and gives a lot of value to anyone who is planning to carry a firearm. Empty your gun and all magazines. Ensure you and a buddy are both completely disarmed with no guns, knives, or other weapons. Place your empty weapon in your holster and demonstrate a common encounter with your buddy. It is then your buddy's job to take your firearm while you are to retain it. There are thousands of different tactics and methods used for weapons retention. However, they all have a common concept: keep your weapon and don't give it up. Start this drill slowly at about 10% speed. The easiest method to retain your weapon is to keep it in its holster, only pulling it out on your terms when you want to. Once you get used to keeping the weapon in the holster forcefully, your buddy can escalate to a higher effort to challenge you more. This drill is designed to illustrate how easy it is for someone to take your weapon and teach you different improvisations you can use to ensure your weapon stays in the holster.

Tactics

1. Cover vs. Concealment

First, we need to understand the difference between cover and concealment. A cover is a hiding place that conceals you from a bad guy and stops bullets. This can be a building, the engine block of a car, a large tree, etc. Concealment is something that hides you but doesn't stop bullets. This can be a bush, the door of a house, a car door, etc. Cover is always preferred to concealment, and it's important to note that it is the only place you should be if you choose to stop moving, like if you need to reload or reassess your situation. Concealment can be used while moving from one place to another tactically, without intending to stay in the same spot for any length of time. A good drill to help practice this concept is simply identifying different structures while you're outside of the home. If you're driving down the road, look at the surrounding areas you pass and think about what you could use for cover and what would be more appropriate as concealment.

2. Tactical Breathing

During intense and high-stress situations (like shootouts or after a physical confrontation), it is common to experience conative delays such as auditory exclusion, tunnel vision, fainting, panic attacks, or hyperventilation. Tactical breathing is a form of *combat meditation* that is commonly taught to the US military and can be used to slightly lower heart rate, defeating these delays and keeping you in the fight. This is accomplished with the four-count principle. First, take in a deep breath while silently counting to four. Next, hold your breath for a second four-count. Finally, exhale while silently counting to four. This 12-second breathing exercise can be repeated until you regain control of your breathing and cognitive ability.

3. Tactical Movement (Walking)

This drill looks funny, but I promise it will prove valuable if you try it as described. First, slightly bend your knees and keep your feet facing straight forward. Begin walking, but roll your feet from heel to toe in an exaggerated style instead of walking with flat feet. This should look and feel funny, but it gets you in the habit of rolling your feet as you move. Continue this for a while to get the hang of it. I recommend walking like this for at least 50 yards. Once you have completed that, draw your firearm and point it in a safe direction, aiming for a small target. Keeping your sight picture on this target, begin walking tactically. You should notice that while you use this method, your sight picture moves much less than if you walked normally. This is tactical movement and when practiced often, will make you travel faster and raise your operational speed.

4. Improvised Weapons

This one is designed to get your mind working in abnormal ways. Look around you at home, work, or out and about, and think about the things in your direct vicinity that you could defend your life with. You need to be realistic about this. Don't say you are going to hit someone with a folding chair if you are sitting in it. Don't say you'll shove something in someone's throat (I don't know why I always hear that during this conversation). Realistically, if someone started killing in the room that you're in, what would you be able to use to defend yourself? You may find that there isn't much for you in this situation, which is by design. If you're not in a place where you have effective improvised weapons readily available, you may want to consider bringing one with you (EDC).

5. Fight to Your Rifle

This is one of my favorite concepts, and it's one that I truly believe in. Know and understand where your final stand is. This is a dark conversation, but it's important to identify it ahead, instead of when you need to. I have always been trained that your hands are used to fight your knife, your knife is used to fight your pistol, and your pistol is used to fight your rifle. I understand this isn't a requirement, but the order makes sense. In extremely close quarters, you may be unable to retrieve even a knife from your belt line to defend yourself. You may be on the ground with someone fighting or cornered against a structure. This is why most martial arts teach to create space. A strike, a throw, or a push that gets a person away from you, creating enough space for you to draw either a knife or a handgun.

The traditional effective use distance for a knife is within 20 feet. If you're within 20 feet, someone can stab you with a knife faster than you can draw a gun and shoot them. "Wait, you said gunfights happen within a few feet." Yes, I did. The traditional 20-foot rule is a scenario-based rule of you vs. them. If someone stools across from you and you both agree that you were going to try to kill each other while within 20 feet, a knife will probably win. However, real self-defense situations are usually sporadic. Usually, someone must be the first to make a move, and they don't stand there and try to intimidate each other like you see in the movies when two people square up to knife fight. It is much more common to see a fistfight escalate into a gun or knife fight. Remember, in a fight, someone must win, and someone must lose, and often the loser doesn't like to accept a loss, so they escalate.

Basic CQB Principles and Tactics

Close Quarters Battle (CQB) is a concept that illustrates tactical strategies and movements to maneuver through a structure or dwelling effectively and quickly. If done properly, CQB movements can keep you safe while also giving you a tactical advantage over your opponent. CQB focuses on body position, angles, structure types, and priority of movement and takes years of practice and repetitions to master.

I want to start by saying that I do not recommend that you attempt these maneuvers or strategies unless you absolutely must. CQB, especially attempted by yourself (Single Person CQB), is dangerous and greatly raises the chances of getting injured or killed in a dynamic situation. These strategies are for educational purposes and should only be used if you are stuck in a dynamic life-and-death situation and you have no other means of solution or escape. Always attempt to remove yourself from a deadly situation without engagement if possible.

As mentioned above, the main elements of CQB are body position, angles, structure types, and movement priority. To understand the basics of CQB is to know how to use these elements together to navigate a building. Many different factors come into play that will challenge these elements. These factors can be time of day (light or dark), location (your home, store, strangers' home), obstacles inside the dwelling, your weapon (long gun or handgun), number of opponents, and if you are alone or with multiple people.

Body Position

The main idea of this element is to ensure that your body is always placed in a position of advantage. If you enter a room, will the bad guy see you before you see them? Are you close enough to the wall that a ricochet that is traveling along the walls could hit you? Are you standing in the center of the room where you can be seen from all other areas? Your goal is to always be within a reasonable distance of cover. That way, if you do take fire, you can have a position that you can get behind to engage your opponent.

Stay out of the middle of the room. Military personnel often call this the "kill zone" because it's where you are most likely to be seen. Stay out of doorways. When entering a room, decide on a direction and commit to it. Standing in a doorway is often called standing in the "fatal funnel." Mainly because there is no place to go, considering the opponent knows you'll be entering the room through that spot. Keep your movement quick but also effective, and travel about 12-18 inches off the walls. Allow your body to act as a turret. Wherever your head looks, your body faces and your gun points at. You should never look at something you are not pointing your gun at in a CQB situation. This is because if you contact an opponent, you do not want to have to reposition yourself to engage them.

Angles

Angles are important because they give you the advantage of seeing more space with less movement. For example, if you are preparing to pass through an area, you can move to the corner of the room and rotate your body to see more of the area. The rule of thumb for most houses in the United States is that if you can see it, you can shoot it. Circular movements and rotations allow you to see more without moving your body into compromised positions. If you choose to enter a room, navigate to the corner of the room while rotating your body, changing the angle of fire, and seeing across the center of the room. This keeps you in an advantaged position while you move and shows you more real estate than if you chose to move laterally. Another good use of angles is when you are traveling down a hallway and passing by doors. If the hallway is narrow, quickly maneuver across from doorways, rotating your upper body while you pass to see as much of the room as possible before committing to moving past it. You can get a better advantage in larger hallways by moving to the opposite side of the hallway from the door. This makes you a smaller target while also allowing you to see more of the room quicker.

A great use of angles is what many in the military call "cutting" or "Slicing the pie." This refers to tactically moving around corners or turning into open spaces. Basically, you line your body up with the corner you are rounding and slowly move in a circular motion around the corner while keeping your weapon fixed to the unknown areas. If done correctly, you should systematically reveal unknown areas one step at a time while limiting the body mass you surrender as a target. This is referred to as slicing the pie because if you do this enough times, your body should move in a complete circle. You remove "pie pieces" of danger areas as you complete this movement.

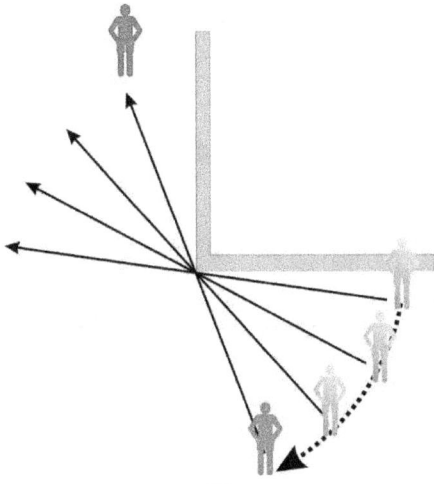

Structure Types

There are thousands of different structure types in the United States and even more diverse structures worldwide. It would not be reasonable to try to train or identify every possible structure type, so the best thing to do is to think conceptually. This can be best achieved by properly addressing standard shapes and building characteristics. One consideration you must address in every structure type is the different styles of room entries. There are corner-fed rooms and there are center-fed rooms. Corner-fed rooms are rooms that have a doorway on the corner, so if you investigate from one side, you will see a wall. If seen from the opposite direction, however, you will find open space and an unknown inside corner that cannot be observed without entering the room in some fashion.

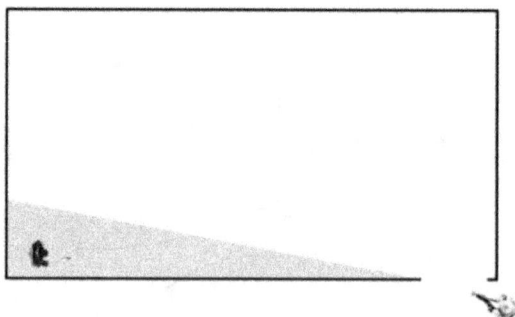

Figure 1. Blind corner of a room.

Using the power of deduction, I'm sure you have figured out that center-fed rooms are rooms that have open areas on both sides because the door is found in the center of a wall and not against a corner. This room creates a new challenge because there will be two unknown inside danger areas that cannot be seen without crossing the threshold of the doorway.

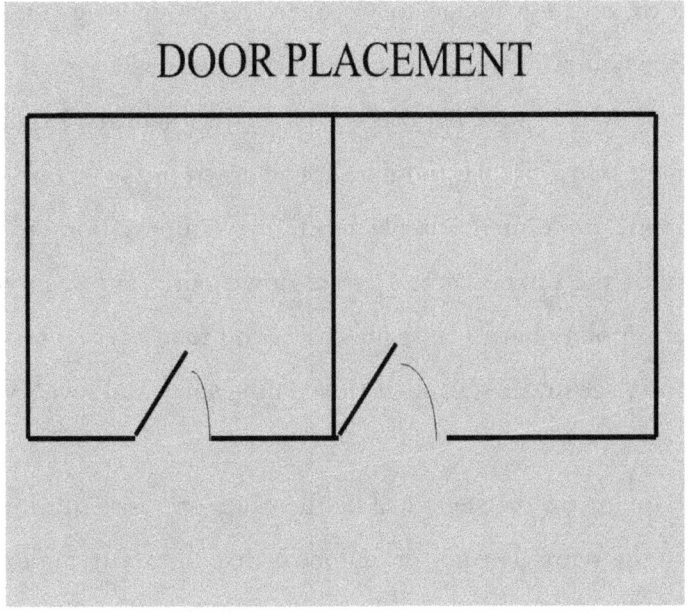

Another structural element you will find in many homes across the country is stairs. Navigating up and down stairs requires different tactics, because you are not only required to use circular angles from left to right, but you must also use up and down angles to maintain a tactical advantage. The best way to tactically navigate stairs is first to try to identify as much of the objective area as possible before positioning yourself on the staircase. For example, if you are traveling down the stairs, try to use as much of the upper level to see all that you can of the lower level. Many homes have balconies that overlook common areas and front entryways. These balconies can be used to your advantage to visualize the lower level prior to putting yourself on the staircase (that is essentially a giant fatal funnel). Once you choose to enter the staircase, quickly navigate it in a circular motion. Travel down the stairs one step at a time while methodically turning your upper body to see more of the unknown real estate downstairs, and keep your firearm pointed at it. In many cases, you may have to crouch down to see under walls that close in the stairs and reveal your legs first.

Moving up the stairs will be the exact opposite of moving down the stairs. The key difference is that you are trying to see as much of the upstairs as you can prior to entering the stairway. Also, you should try to use the open area to visualize any existing balconies, doorways, and common areas that may be at the top. Once you are on the stairs, move up the steps one at a time while using your upper body like a turret, methodically turning to see the unknown area as you continue advancing.

It is important to note that you should not be navigating up or down stairs unless you have completely cleared the level you are on or unless you are attempting to make a quick escape. Stairs can also be used immediately if you know for a fact that the opponent is not on the same floor as you are currently.

Priority of Movement

All your CQB movements should be completed according to tactical priority. This essentially means that you are addressing the most danger first. For example, if you are navigating a hallway and see open and closed doors, the priority would be to open doors. This is because the closed doors add an additional layer of safety (and danger) for you or an opponent to overcome prior to a possible engagement. While conducting your movements, you can determine the priority for your travel direction based on indicators and stimuli. Indicators are physical identifiers that tell you what is happening inside a certain area. These can be blood, bullets, broken furniture or glass, bodies, or disheveled items. A stimulus, however, is most often a sound. Good examples of a stimulus are gunshots, talking or screaming, furniture or property shuffling, footsteps, or anything abnormal.

If you are in a dynamic situation and are trying to get away, you would listen for stimuli like gunshots or screaming and go in the opposite direction. You would also use indicators if no stimulus were present. If you are in a situation at your home, such as a home invasion, you would listen for footsteps, whispering, and the general sounds of looting. You would also look for indicators such as broken glass, flashlights, and shadows, and you will choose which direction you travel based on these elements.

Recommended Combat Drills

Of all the combat drills, and there are thousands, many are focused on specific movements, strategies, and/or skills. While this is okay (better something than nothing), I would argue that cognitive training is the best training a beginner can do. Purposefully placing oneself under pressure to simulate the effects of combat within a safe training environment. I call this cognitive training not because it's a mental exercise but because your body will react differently when pressure is applied. For example, if you are someone who goes to the gun range and shoots holes in a paper target (we already talked about that), you probably won't perform at your peak potential in combat. I would sooner trade that training for running sprints and changing magazines between runs. Maybe do some pushups until your arms give out, then try to shoot the same piece of paper. I would confidently guess that your shot groups would be much less consistent.

Cognitive training doesn't have to be for just shooting, either. Applying stress to your normal drilling activities will absolutely make you more adept at those responses. If you are practicing your "fire drills," try doing them quickly while also having to save a loved one. For example, you can fill a duffel bag with books to simulate a child and attempt to safely and tactically leave your house to avoid a home invader or a house fire. Adding extra elements of pressure or stress will force you to improvise and adapt to the situation, making you more prepared for the unknown. One of the best pieces of advice I ever heard was told to me as a child when I was learning to ride a bike. I was in a gravel parking lot, complaining that it was hard because the rocks were making the tires slide under me. I was told that if I could learn to ride a bike well on gravel, imagine how easy it would be on a flat road. This resonated with me for the rest of my life, and I have been able to apply this to most hardships in my life. If I must reload my rifle under pressure while only using one hand, imagine how easy it will be normally. If I must finish this college paper after a long day of work while also taking care of my kids, imagine how easy it would be normally. This may sound like romanticizing hindsight, but it helps me be better at difficult tasks and appreciate the results I earn.

This concept is not new. Some of the nation's most elite groups train this way. It's been proven that adding stress to a training simulation makes it more valuable training. This is why Navy Seals train against the waves of the ocean. It's why Marines spar dynamically with each other while learning hand-to-hand combat. It's why Air Force pilots simulate flight at the highest altitudes, often causing them to lose consciousness. It's why the Army spends months getting screamed at by drill sergeants to complete even the simplest tasks. Pressure is what's required to create diamonds. The pressure pushes you to your *real* limits. Pressure will make you dangerous.

Basic Spontaneous Knife Defense

I want to preface this section by laying out a very real disclaimer and standard. If you find yourself in a situation where you are faced with a person armed with a knife, escape is the absolute best option, if possible. If you choose to attempt to engage someone with a knife physically, you are almost certain to get cut. In this book, you will not learn or be encouraged to knife fight or learn any of the ninja moves you see in action movies and from the high-speed operators on YouTube. The harsh reality is that the best way to win a knife fight is to avoid it at all costs. This includes all edged and pointed weapons.

The first basic rule of spontaneous knife defense is to put space and obstacles between you and your opponent. If someone is trying to cut you and you run to the other side of your car, you can run in circles with him/her until help arrives. Create space as quickly as possible and look for something wide enough that you can't be touched from the other side. While this is happening, be loud. Scream that you're being attacked, scream that he/she has a knife, and scream loudly so that everyone can hear. The chances are that either someone will help or call for help, or the person will not like the attention and will flee the area. While I understand this is not sexy, it is the best way to keep yourself alive if someone is trying to attack you with an edged weapon.

If, for whatever reason, you are trapped and cannot flee from the assailant, you *must* prioritize controlling the weapon. The first step is to isolate it. This can be accomplished by controlling someone's wrist with your full attention while they are holding the blade. Both hands on one to ensure you have physical superiority. Next, create leverage. Typically, you'll want to do this with a hard object, like a car, a light pole, a door frame, etc. You'll take the arm that has the knife and ram it violently into the edge of one of these objects, targeting the forearm. This should either break the arm or shock the nerves enough to make them drop the weapon.

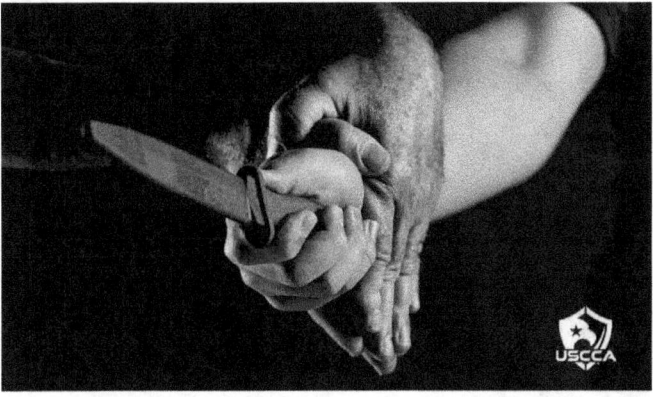

Keep in mind this isn't about self-defense at this point; it's about survival. You will probably be assaulted, punched, kicked, bitten, scratched, and whatever else they can do to get that knife back in the fight. Your movements must be rapid, violent, and objective. Once the knife is out of the attacker's hand, do not try to recover it. This is a good opportunity to flee the area. If this is still impossible, create space between the attacker and the knife. You don't recover it because if it is not in anyone's possession, it isn't a factor in the fight. If you possess it, there is always a chance you could lose that possession and return to fighting for your life.

A very effective (and fun) way to practice knife defense is to buy a pack of white shirts and a couple of sharpies. Have a friend, coworker, spouse, etc., try to mark your shirt with the sharpie, and you try to keep it clean. If you get a marker on the shirt, that is the equivalent to a cut. Simple but effective, and this training will also demonstrate how incredibly difficult it is to defend yourself from an edged weapon. Finally, the best way to train to beat a knife is with a gun. If you are training properly and choose to carry a firearm every day, this scenario changes slightly.

If a knife is pulled, your objective is still to make space, put an object between you and the assailant, and attempt to flee. However, should this not be possible, you can now focus on drawing your firearm instead of attempting to disarm your attacker. This is done by creating as much space as possible. Note also that your gun should not come out unless space can be made. Once your gun leaves the holster, it is not an element of the fight, and it can potentially be used for you or against you.

To train for this scenario, have your empty and unloaded gun in the holster with no magazines inserted. Have your friend with the sharpie try to mark your white shirt again, except this time, elude them to make space and draw your gun before they can get to you. This type of training can be very fun but also teach you some valuable skills. Like everything in this book, the more you practice and train, the more proficient you will become.

Reacting to an Active Shooter

What is an Active Shooter?

Knowing the difference between an active shooter and a shooting is important. These incidents require different responses, and you must understand what to do in these situations. An active shooter is a person who's actively shooting people inside a target-rich environment. Keep in mind, I said *actively,* which means continuously shooting multiple people and haven't stopped. An active shooter is a dynamic incident that is still happening in real time.

Psychology of a Rampage Killer

There have been thousands of studies on active shooters, rampage killers, and other crazies that want to hurt large numbers of people. One of the most consistent things in these studies is the inconsistencies. The fact of the matter is that rampage killers are illogical. They choose to kill many people as fast as they can so they can send a message. Unfortunately, with the state of the media in the United States, active shooter situations are very publicized and place the maniac in the spotlight where they want to be. Notice that a lot of rampage killers release manifestos or blogs prior to their mass killings. This is more than likely because they know that it will be released nationwide if they kill a lot of people. If they didn't, it would just be another person bitching on the internet that gets ignored.

Rampage killers know they are going to be killed. They assume that this will be their last day on earth and choose to take out as many people as possible because their message is worth their life. It is also interesting to note that while many rampage killers release videos and manifestos if they fail to die and are caught, they remain suspiciously quiet. I won't pretend I know why this is, but I would venture to guess that it's because they know they failed their mission. These people want to kill and then die. Giving them verbal commands will not stop them. Telling them about your wife and kids will not help. They cannot show empathy, and are more invested in their mission and message than in their emotions.

If you find yourself in a situation where you are near an active shooter, you have a decision to make. If you are armed, is it your duty to defend the others in the area? Do you have family or loved ones with you? Ultimately, the decision is yours, and you'll be the one who must live with it. Since this book is just a beginner guide, I will focus on being unarmed and reacting to this type of incident.

<u>Get Away</u>

The first thing to do in this situation is to get away from the shooting. This seems obvious, but I want you to focus on making this a long-term solution. First, you should see if there is an immediate way out of the building or area. Chances are the killer will not leave the area because that's where all the people (targets) are. If there is no immediate means of escape, begin the process of moving away from the stimulus. If you see a large group of people running into another room, that may be the next place the shooter chooses (target-rich environment). If possible, find a spot that may be difficult to get into or out of, even though that may sound counterproductive. Rampage killers are on the clock, and their mission is to rack up a kill count as quickly as they can before they are killed. They are not likely to try to fight heavily fortified areas, multiple locks, barricades, or tight and small spaces. They will likely move on and try to find targets they can reach quickly.

Try to find a room with a lock on the door, get inside, and start barricading it. If no such room exists, find a small place to hide, like a closet under a pile of clothes, a cabinet under a counter, or even a storage box or container. This seems foolish, but if you're looking for a large group of people, you probably won't find them in a box.

Fortify Your Area

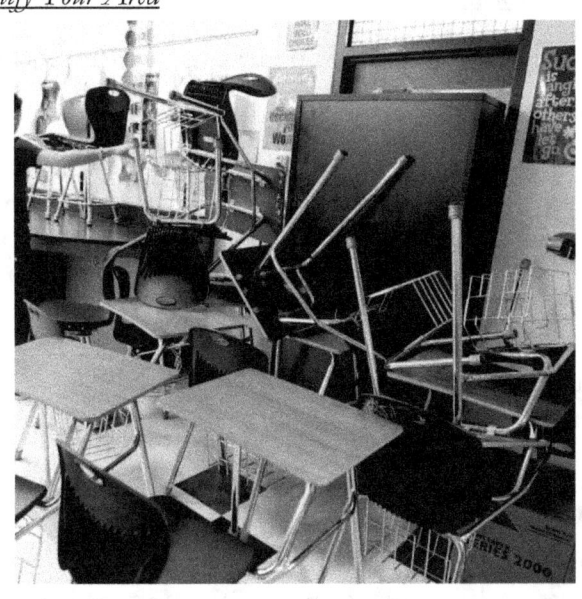

Once you find your spot, the next action you must take is fortifying. Barricade the door and make it as difficult for a bad guy to get into. If you are in a classroom, this can be done using a method called "Small, Large, Small." Close and lock the door. Jam door stoppers, wood, books, etc., under the door, to make it harder to open. Place a chair under the doorknob at an angle to reinforce the barricade. Next, find the heaviest furniture at your disposal and begin to pile it against the door, completely covering the door, the door frame, and any windows that may be near it. Once that is finished, turn out the lights and hide inside the room to the best of your ability. No one except the police should open the door.

Defend Yourself

If you find that you have no means of fortification and you are at risk of being contacted by the shooter, do not panic. Come up with a plan for when the contact will occur and communicate it to anyone who may be with you. Plan to fight for your life and assume victory. Find something that can be used as an impact or edged weapon. This could be a broomstick, a table leg, or a piece of broken glass. Something that you would be afraid of if being threatened with it. Stage yourself in an area of opportunity. Pay attention to the killer's location and the direction they will likely approach you from. Position yourself so they cannot see you immediately, giving yourself the element of surprise. Lower your level by crouching or taking a knee. A shooter will more than likely be shooting at people who are running and standing and most likely will not be thinking about someone who is crouched down. When you finally see the killer, do not hesitate, do not wait, do not try to speak to them. Attack with your strongest blows at their most vital areas (head, neck, groin, face) and continue the assault until the person is no longer a threat. This sounds barbaric and primitive, but remember that they put themselves in this situation and expect to be killed. If a rampage killer with a wish to die tries to harm me, I will ensure they get their wish.

Post Incident Notes

A few things need to be mentioned about this type of incident that are often overlooked by trainers but are very important. First, if you must get physical with the attacker, do not stay near them. Attack them swiftly and violently until they are no longer a threat, then attempt again to get away. Keep in mind the only more dangerous thing than the shooter is the police who are attempting to find the shooter. Often, law enforcement does not have an accurate description of the killer, if they have one at all. Also, many agencies will discontinue radio communications during an incident like this to avoid the likelihood of detonating explosives that may be in the area. Therefore, being present and covered in blood in an area where the shooter was last seen with a weapon near you is a recipe for getting shot by the police. Get away from the area and link up with law enforcement peacefully later.

Also, understand that you were just involved in a dynamic incident. You will not remember everything that has occurred in full detail, and you may not be able to give an accurate statement to the police. To avoid perjuring yourself or giving a false statement, refrain from speaking to law enforcement for a few days. Police should understand if they are properly trained. However, in my experience, many are not.

Finally, make sure you go to the hospital. Even if you weren't shot, you must seek medical attention. You may have broken a bone, torn a muscle, or even sustained internal damage that you aren't able to feel due to the influx of adrenalin in your body. If left unchecked, these injuries could worsen in the following days.

Basic Self-Defense Tactics

This book would almost certainly fail if I didn't at least break into a few different methods of defending yourself in a dynamic physical confrontation. While there are literally *thousands* of disciplines, techniques, and strategies to study and master in this category, I will focus primarily on simplicity and basics that will save your life. These tactics are violent by design and require speed without hesitation. Remember, when it's your life on the line against an assailant, there is no referee and no fouls. To start, I want to get into unarmed conflict. This is important for you to understand to lay a foundation for you to use more advanced tactics. The moves listed below demonstrate just that.

<u>Eye Jab</u>

A classic target for defending yourself, often referred to as "the groin of the face" is the eyes. It truly does not matter if you're a black belt martial artist or a 500lb bodybuilder; a shot to the eyes will impair you. The main idea of this move is not to "poke" necessarily but more to *rake the eyes*. Create a claw shape with your hand and swipe horizontally across the face. We rake and do not poke because eyes are a small target. The goal is to create the greatest possibility of an accurate strike to the eyes and not missing to poke someone in the forehead.

Headbutt

I always tell my peers never to underestimate the power of a good headbutt. A headbutt is an effective move because it's rarely telegraphed, and the assailant probably won't see it coming. This is a great option if you are in close quarters, such as a bear hug or attacking in a tight space. The goal is to strike in a forward ramming-style motion instead of a whipping motion. Using the crown of the skull, approximately two inches above your hairline, ram the central part of the face. Aiming for the nose is an easy target, and even if you miss a little, the orbital bone, eyes, and mouth may still be struck, allowing you to get away.

Throat Chop/ Punch

Attacking the throat is a great way to immobilize an attacker, giving you room to flee or get to a weapon. There are delicate spots in the throat, including the corraded artery, the esophagus, and the larynx. Please note that an attack on any of these areas with enough force can potentially cause death. Therefore, it should be reserved only for dire circumstances where you fear for your life. In the position where a punch is easier, be sure to punch straight forward, targeting right below the chin. If you miss and hit the chin, there is a good chance you could still immobilize them. If your attacker is sideways, you may consider a chop to the corraded, located on the side of the neck. Aim approximately an inch or two under the ear, and be sure to keep the strike above the collarbone and shoulder. This strike can also affect the brachial plexus origin, creating the possibility to stun the attacker for five to seven seconds. Any strike to the neck also has a possibility of damaging the spine or brainstem if struck hard enough or if using an impact weapon.

Kicking / Attacking the Groin

This one has become a well-known standard, and despite being almost expected, it is still a very viable and effective defense technique. The groin is one of the more vulnerable places on a person's body, especially a male. That's why attacking that area will elicit a response every time. Remember, attacking doesn't just have to be a kick. A punch, or knee, or elbow will be just as effective. Use whatever you can to generate a large amount of energy to impact that area, and you'll be able to disable the attacker long enough to flee.

Attack the Knee

This one isn't as popular; however, it is very effective. Attacking someone's knee is a great way to disable them and achieve a safe retreat. This attack can be used without much telegraphing by "sparta-kicking" the kneecap in a forward stomping motion. This will hyper-extend the knee, potentially breaking bones, tearing muscles and ligaments, throwing the attacker off balance, and ultimately disabling them. This move is not fatal, but it is very damaging and has the potential for a psychological factor should the assailant see his leg at an odd angle.

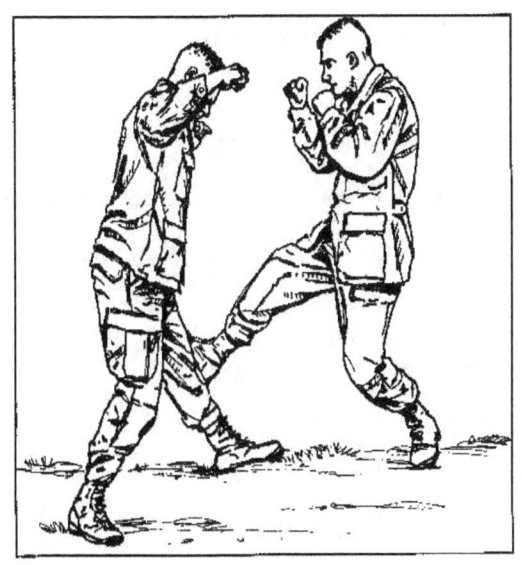

Urban Survival Tactics

Survival in an urban environment is a very important topic to a dangerous person. I use the word survival here because simply identifying one or two threats in this demographic will not suffice. In the spirit of being dangerous, you need to be well-rounded and truly understand what to look for and what actions to take while navigating through dangerous areas. Since we have already discussed risk mitigation tactics, this section will focus on proactive measures to help you thrive in an Urban environment where danger is present.

Blending

You may notice that this topic has already been mentioned in this book, and you are correct. This is mentioned again because it will be a little different this time. Urban environments come with unique risks and a different culture to be aware of. One very important aspect of blending is to not look like you're out of your element. Often, people who visit New York City are victimized because, little do they know, they stick out like a sore thumb.

Don't look up at the high sky-scraper buildings while you are walking around. This is tourist behavior and will quickly label you as a target. Keep your head down or straight ahead, and leave your phone and wallet in your pockets with your hands down. Also, do not walk while looking at your phone. Staying alert and vigilant is vital when moving through such densely populated areas.

If you find that you are in an urban area when danger is present (riot, shootings, terror attack, etc.), the first thing to do is to attempt to blend with the environment around you. This means that if people are running around fire-bombing stores with their shirts off, you should take your shirt off as well. This will buy time while you seek an exit from the area without looking out of place. The next step will be to find a smaller group of people who are moving away and attach yourself to them. There is power in numbers, and groups of people are not targeted as much as people who are alone. You don't have to interact or speak to them, just walk near them as you exit the area. Finally, do not get into a vehicle while you're still in danger. Blocking roads and surrounding vehicles has become a common practice in riots and leaves you little opportunity to escape safely.

Consider dressing in layers in an urban environment. This is a good practice for a few reasons, but mostly because it allows you to change your appearance if you need to quickly. For example, if you find that you are caught in a dangerous situation and must fight to get away, there is a good chance that you will be pursued. Dressing in layers will allow you to strip clothing once you are out of sight to avoid re-detection. Ensure that you immediately change your trajectory and demeanor if you do this. If you are sprinting south and round a corner, shedding your jacket, the next thing to do would be to turn again and begin walking like you are not involved in whatever that person running was doing.

Every Day Carry

If you happen to live in an urban environment, your EDC considerations may differ from those living in more rural areas. EDC of a firearm in an urban environment should represent your daily actions. For example, if you take a subway every day, you should consider carrying your firearm in an appendix holster to not have a chance of your gun being against a passenger sitting beside you. Another good idea would be to have a wallet and a money clip. Hear me out: if you are robbed at gunpoint, the safest thing to do is comply (if only briefly) with the robber's demands. Providing a money clip with a few dollars saves them from obtaining your cards and ID, which also has your personal information and address on it. I am not suggesting that the robber getaway, but sometimes a distraction or deflection can create a perfect opportunity for you to act.

Responding to Chaos

It's no secret that urban environments will be among the first to be targeted for a mass attack. This could be anything from an active shooter to an act of terror. We know that this is done because of the dense population and the mass media coverage the attack will receive. It's crucial to understand what it takes to survive this type of situation and get away unscathed.

The first thing to do is determine if escape is possible. If you are on the outskirts of the incident and can leave the area, that is a priority. If you find that you are at ground zero and you haven't been medically disabled by injury, your next move is to seek shelter. Don't think of shelter as a house but as a place that can shield you from another attack. Look for a place that is isolated from large groups of people and doesn't have the immediate appearance of safety. For example, this could be a car wash, a laundry mat, or even a dumpster. Something you can get inside that is not likely to have many people in it.

Once you have found your shelter, it's time for you to double-check for wounds and injuries. It is very possible that if you were wounded, the adrenaline of the incident would cause you to be unaware. Take your hand in a bear-claw shape, and systematically rake your skin from the top of your head, working down your torso. Be sure to be thorough and get under your arms and in your groin. It's important to keep your hand in a rake shape to ensure that you 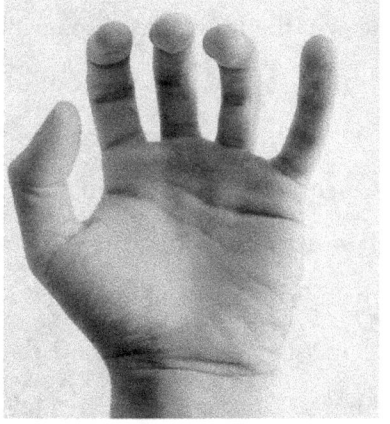 aren't wiping blood but instead feeling for cuts and holes. After each section (head, neck, upper body, lower body) look at your hands to see if there is blood. This will help you isolate and determine where the injury is should one exist.

If you are injured, apply pressure directly to the wound to stop the bleeding. If it is a serious wound, ball up some cloth from a shirt or sock and place it directly on the wound. Next, tie the other sock or shirt sleeve around the wound tightly, if possible. The chances are that your cell phone will be useless due to the volume of calls that will inevitably go out during this incident, but you can use it for the GPS function to map the best route out of the area.

Next, you need to walk, if possible. Once you have determined the immediate attack has concluded, you need to leave the area (on foot if possible). Waiting on rescue efforts to win the immediate area will likely take hours, if not days, to get aid to you. Walking out of the area and going even a mile out of the way could get you immediate medical attention. Once again, avoid getting into a vehicle for as long as possible. It is *very* likely that all surrounding roadways will be closed, making it impossible for you to move in any capacity other than on foot. If you find that you have a broken leg or an injured foot, consider stealing a bicycle. I know this decision feels odd, but as described in the morals vs. ethics section, we make decisions that will keep us alive. You can ride a bike with only one foot, and it will allow you to get out of the area. Urban areas typically have many bike riders, and there will almost certainly be one somewhere around you.

The Zombie Apocalypse – The Final Test

One of my favorite topics is the Zombie Apocalypse. What will I do, where will I go, and who will I have on my ZA team? It's a fun way to theorize and strategize for disaster while also testing your readiness. When I think of the zombie apocalypse, however, I don't think of brain-eating undead humanoids who hoard up and infect anything that moves. Instead, I think of mass panic. Everyone else is a "Zombie" in my scenario because everyone else is also trying to survive this disaster. Civil unrest, government tyranny, politically charged riots, or even natural disasters. In all reality, we have seen small examples of the ZA already.

Domestic Acts of Terror

I still remember 9/11 very well, and although I was just a child, what stood out to me most was the impact it had on everyone, even those who were across the nation. Domestic Terror is something that is used as a tool to create fear. These acts are usually done by bombing, spreading weaponized illness, or using dangerous improvised weapon devices. Although most Americans immediately think of 9/11 when they hear "terror." I like to think of smaller-scale massacres because I feel like there is a much greater chance of them happening again. For example, the Boston Marathon bombing, where an improvised explosive device made from a pressure cooker was used to kill and cause great bodily injury to dozens of athletes and spectators. Typically, targets will include a target-rich environment that may be highly visible to the public (TV, radio, internet streaming) and may have the possibility of having important people present.

Natural Disaster/ Hurricane Katrina

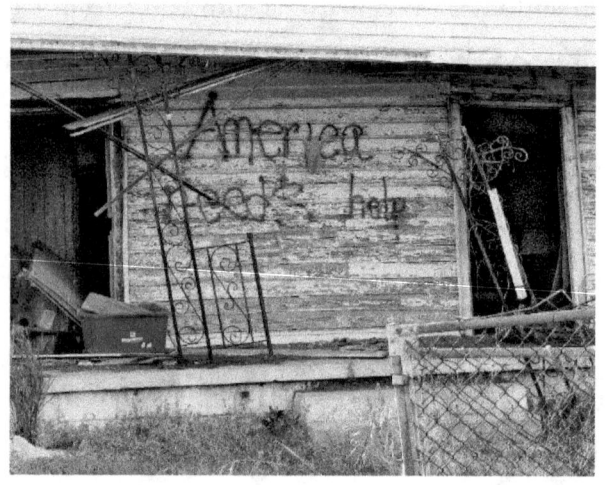

In 2005, Hurricane Katrina rolled through New Orleans, destroying everything in her path and creating the need for a panicked response from the people who lived there. Mass panic, looting, violence, and forced survival were caused by slow or even no immediate rescue efforts and people fearing for their lives. Nearly 1/3 of law enforcement had fled the city prior to Katrina's arrival, and roadblocks were put in place on the city limits, quarantining citizens in place to limit the area requiring reestablished governance. There were areas of prolonged flooding, causing dangerous conditions such as limiting food and potable water, limiting travel options, and even potential health risks like dehydration, food poisoning, and spreading disease. All these factors combined bear a staggering resemblance to what many would imagine a zombie apocalypse would be like.

Protests/ Riots

It was almost a standard for a while: a police officer abuses their power, a politician makes an unpopular statement, or a large corporation gets greedy. The response is usually to have a protest that will ultimately turn into a riot. This includes burning down a convenience store, looting and destroying businesses and property, and creating chaos. Cars get flipped, small businesses get torched, and police officers get abused. For the average person, this should be terrifying. Not only does this jeopardize your family's safety, and makes it nearly impossible to live a normal life in that geographical area. Considering the long-term effects of civil unrest will promptly reveal damage to the economy due to the inevitable closure of small businesses and devastating loss of infrastructure and inventory, there will more than likely be a spike in crime as well. This fits into the model of a zombie apocalypse due to the potential danger you will encounter within the immediate area.

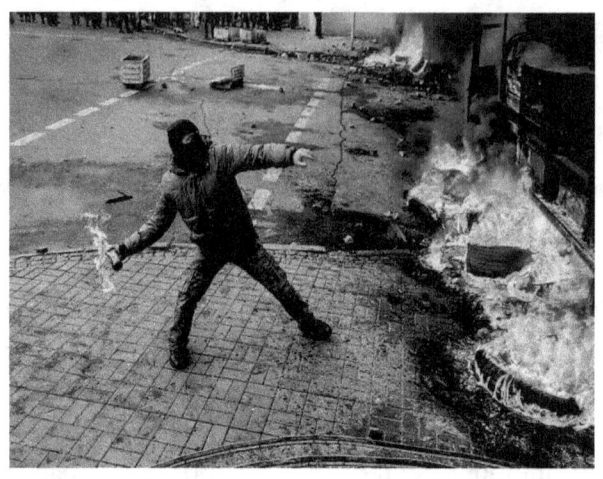

Pandemic/ Mass Illnesses

COVID-19 had a massive effect on the world. The United States was also impacted by our liberties during the pandemic due to many people resisting quarantine protocols, failing to abide by mask mandates, and refusing vaccination recommendations. Ultimately, your position on these topics is still a heated and controversial area of debate, even years later. This led Americans to question the integrity of the government and the possibility of fear-mongering. Those on the other side of the coin vocalized the frustrations of those who did not follow protocols, potentially worsening the illness. Regardless of your position on this topic, this is a perfect example of a "zombie apocalypse" because it contains a biological threat, the threat of tyranny, and the possibility of civil war.

Why is this information relevant to being dangerous? One aspect of danger is being able to forecast and proactively respond to threats. Suppose you can foresee an incident of civil unrest. In that case, you may be able to fortify your home, prepare your family, and even secure precious supplies before they become scarce commodities due to panic buying, looting, and damage. Maybe you plan to "bug out" leaving behind your property and material possessions to seek a better, more secure environment.

On the other hand, maybe you believe that "digging in" is the better option and choose to fortify your home, stock bulk supplies, create sustainable resources, and defend your property as the storm passes. Without the proper information, appropriately making this decision is almost impossible. For example, you may plan to bug out because you romanticize exactly what it entails without considering what that entails. Or maybe you plan to dig in, even though a natural disaster is almost a certain defeat of your property and everything surrounding it.

Conclusion

You shouldn't attribute to malice what can more than likely be attributed to incompetence. Most people aren't on a mission to hurt you. The fact of the matter is that most people are living in their own world as the *star* of their own story. It's up to you to stay alert and recognize the people who want to be the *villain* in your story. Being dangerous is a mindset, a lifestyle, and, most importantly, a choice.

You are responsible for your safety. You cannot rely on others to protect you from imminent danger while sacrificing their own safety. Though many law enforcement officers, military personnel, agents from alphabet soup agencies, and prior service members will gladly step up and answer the call, you can't be willing to bet your life on it. Take the initiative by training passionately with intensity and progressively greater challenges. Prepare for the worst, although you're hoping for the best. Always strive to be the most dangerous person in the room. Turn these practices into habits and the habits into lifestyle, and you may find it saves your life one day…

About the Author

Jonathan Von Moltke is a United States Army Veteran, and served as a Psychological Operations Specialist (37F) before being honorably discharged after completion of his eight-year contract. He was a law enforcement officer in South Carolina for over a decade and also worked in roles such as uniformed patrol, warrants, SWAT operations, SRT command, criminal investigations, homicide investigative response, undercover operations, law enforcement training, advanced law enforcement training, and administrative command. Jonathan has earned South Carolina state-level certifications in basic instructor training, specific skills instructor, firearms instructor, defensive tactics instructor, field training officer, field training officer manager, training manager, and was federally certified as an instructor in active shooter threat response through the Department of Homeland Security (FLETC). Jonathan is a competitive marksman and have studied multiple disciplines of martial arts, combatives, and combat sports. He is a hobbyist for survival and disaster preparation and continuously seeks new ways to stay proficient and prepared for danger.

www.ingramcontent.com/pod-product-compliance
Lightning Source LLC
Chambersburg PA
CBHW050202130526
44591CB00034B/1969